ACKNOWLEDGEMENTS

I would like to thank Gillian Sturgess for initiating this book, Dr Ian Banks and Karen Evennett for help with parts of the text, and Paul Smith for being such a patient editor.

CONTENTS

T'CTC

Dr

UNIVERSITY OF
GLOUCESTERSHIRE
at Cheltenham and Gloucester

Copyright © 1994 Alan Maryon Davis

British Library Cataloguing in Publication Data

Maryon Davis, Alan
Good Health Guide
I. Title
613

ISBN 1 85448 987 9 (paperback)

First published 1994
Illustrations by Christine Roche
Typeset by Type Generation Ltd, Lond
Printed in England

Health Education Authority
Hamilton House
Mabledon Place
London WC1H 9TX

INTRODUCTION

With all the health advice that's flying about these days, on the TV and radio, and in the magazines and papers, you could be forgiven for thinking that enough is enough and you'd just like to be left to get on with your life.

The trouble is that not all the advice is sound or sensible. The media thrive on controversy, and happily give lots of coverage to anyone with something different to say, to whoever wants to rock the boat, or who's just plain whacky. The latest crackpot wonder-diet, a new device for exercising without effort, the scientist who claims that cholesterol is good for you, a pH-balanced skin formula to banish wrinkles, 100 easy ways to achieve orgasm – you know the sort of thing - the list is virtually endless. Fascinating though it all is, it can be very confusing. You could very easily get the impression that doctors can't even agree amongst themselves about what constitutes a healthy diet, or what's the best way to get fit, or whether there's such a thing as stress. You might even be tempted to ignore the lot of them and just carry on the same way you always have.

But that would be a great shame, because the good news is that there's actually a wealth of solid scientific evidence from around the world showing that the right balance of foods, combination of activities, or avoidance of damaging influences, can make a huge difference to your health, not only in twenty or thirty years' time, but also right now – today or tomorrow or next week.

Even better news is the fact that, far from being boring, if you go about it the right way, healthy living can be positively enjoyable. It can actually be fun to keep in shape. And you'll get much more joy out of life if you're looking and feeling good.

That's the essential message I've tried to convey in this book. It needn't be difficult to help yourself to better health. And it certainly shouldn't be irksome or miserable. If that's the way you see it at the moment, then I do hope the following chapters will persuade you otherwise.

I've tried to gather together in this slim volume as many of the basic facts and pieces of straightforward practical advice as I can. I've tried to answer the questions most people ask about healthy eating, physical activity, stress and relaxation, sleep, smoking, alcohol, drugs, sex, women's health, and health for older people. And, where possible, I've summarised the essential points for easy reference.

So, over to you. I do hope you'll take up the challenge. Why not make a fresh start right now? In easy stages – just a minor change here and there at first – but building up slowly to a whole new way of living.

Good luck and good health!

Alan Maryon Davis

EATING FOR LIFE

The good news

For most of us, eating is more than a mere means of survival – it's also one of life's great pleasures. Fortunately, as far as our health is concerned, the good news is that healthy eating doesn't have to mean boring eating. Far from it. Scientific evidence from around the world has shown that the everyday diets that help to protect against such major killers as heart disease and cancer are varied and delicious combinations of good, wholesome foods.

The not-so-good news

But the not-so-good news is that far too many of us have got ourselves into a rut of unhealthy eating – day in, day out – year in, year out. High fat snacks, chocolate bars, deep fried foods, fatty burgers, chips with everything, washed down with sugary drinks – the list of ever-available temptations is a long one. And it isn't just children who are hooked on these things – many adults are too, especially men. It's partly habit, partly convenience, partly price and partly lack of awareness or imagination.

This is a great shame because a glance round any supermarket will prove that, more than ever before, we have an incredible range of wonderful foods from which to choose. With so many people taking holidays abroad, developing a liking for the local cuisine, and so many different cultures now part of our multi-ethnic society, our high streets are brimming with a cornucopia of exciting, exotic delicacies.

There's no doubt that we have much to learn from each other's traditional national diet. Everyday eating in some countries is distinctly healthier than in others. Just within Europe, for example, we now know that countries bordering on the Mediterranean have much lower rates of heart disease than those in northern Europe, including Britain. Why should that be? The evidence suggests that it is the Mediterranean combination of fresh fruit, lightly cooked vegetables, pasta or rice, fish, chicken, olive oil, garlic, and a fondness for wine, that has a more beneficial effect on the heart than the red meat and dairy based diets of countries further north.

What's wrong with our diet?

As a nation, we eat too much fatty food, too much sugary food, too much salty food, and not enough fibre-rich starchy food and vitamin-laden fruit. And there's a very long list of ills that are lying in wait for us as a result. Here are the main threats to our health:

- **Coronary heart disease**
  Angina and heart attacks are caused by silting up of the coronary arteries in the heart with a fatty substance, cholesterol. This, in turn, is largely determined by our consumption of fatty foods, especially those high in saturated fats – mainly meat, sausages, pies, and full-fat dairy products.

- **Strokes**
  The result of damage to one of the arteries supplying the brain, strokes are often linked to high blood pressure. This, in turn, is more likely to affect people who eat a lot of salt, drink a lot of alcohol, or are overweight.

- **Diabetes**
  Overweight people are more likely to develop diabetes in middle age. This can cause a number of health problems, including heart disease.

- **Bowel problems**
  Insufficient dietary fibre (mainly due to a lack of fibre-rich starchy foods, vegetables and fruit) is linked to constipation and a number of bowel diseases, such as piles, diverticular disease and bowel cancer.

- **Tooth decay and gum disease**
  Eating or drinking too many sugary things encourages mouth bacteria (plaque) to produce acid, which destroys tooth enamel and irritates gums.

- **Obesity**
  Apart from increasing the risk of heart disease, stroke and diabetes, an excess of body-fat is likely to aggravate such conditions as back-ache, arthritis, foot problems, and gallstones. It also increases the risk of post-operative complications after surgery. The most calorie-packed foods or drinks are those loaded with fat (or oil), sugar or alcohol.

The new awareness

There's no doubt that most people are much more aware of the healthy eating message than they used to be. Magazines and TV programmes have been pushing the basic rules for a long time. There's much more interest now in choosing and preparing food than there was even a few years ago.

But some people are worried that they may not be able to afford a healthy diet. Those on low incomes – lone parents, pensioners, unemployed people – may be convinced that healthier alternatives are more expensive. In fact, dietitians' opinions differ on this, but all agree that it needn't cost any more to make some really significant improvements in your or your family's diet. Switching to semi-skimmed milk, for example; wholemeal bread rather than white; chicken instead of red meat; more starchy staples like potatoes, beans or rice; lots of greens, carrots, and onions; low-sugar, low-salt cereals; cutting the fat off meat; more fruit in season; fewer processed or pre-cooked meals – these simple changes needn't be costly – indeed they could even save you money.

In this chapter, we'll look at why changing to a healthier everyday diet is so important, and how it can make life more, not less, pleasurable.

STAYING SLIM

The overweight epidemic

Nobody wants to be flabby, and we all know it's unhealthy - yet, according to recent surveys, fatness has never been more popular. In Britain, for example, four out of ten men, and about three out of ten women, are overweight. In some other developed countries – notably the United States, Australia and Germany – the proportion of tubbies is even higher.

Why is that? Why, despite a multi-million dollar slimming industry, pushing every conceivable diet, exercise programme and cellulite-dissolving potion, are so many of us so fat? And getting fatter.

Perhaps the real reason is that 'going on a diet', or tackling this or that bulging contour, is missing the most fundamental point. Perhaps instead we should con-centrate on what is natural for the human body, and change our everyday pattern of eating and exercising to something closer to the one the human body has naturally evolved.

The human race originated as hunter-gatherers in the great grasslands of the old African land mass. Our diet was a mixture of many different foods, mostly of plant origin – roots, shoots, grains and fruits – and occasionally meat from animals trapped or speared. Some who lived near rivers, lakes or seas also ate fish and molluscs.

It was a diet largely of fibre-rich starchy foods which provided most of the bulk and energy we needed. Obtaining the food used up almost as much energy as we gained by eating it. Life was hard – and very few of us were fat.

Nowadays, in the developed world, although we still have essentially the same human body, we have lost this balance with Nature. We have gone soft. Our diet is aeons away from the one we were designed to eat. And the only hunting and gathering most of us do is in search of the nearest take-away.

The result is that we're suffering an epidemic of obesity the like of which we've never seen before, and we search in vain for a wonder-breakthrough diet magically to vanish away our spare tyres and horrible hips and thighs.

Gorging for comfort

Eating, quite simply, provides pleasure and comfort. When we eat, brain hormones called endorphins induce a feeling of pleasure and contentment. In times of stress, or when we are feeling down or lacking in confidence, a good feed makes things seem a whole lot better – at least for a while. Then we look in the mirror and see a bulging, bulbous, flabby creature that refuses to fit into our clothes and we feel bad all over again.

How fat is fat?

Most people who are overweight know about it – although some, especially men, may not be very prepared to admit it to themselves. Certainly, if you're a woman, the chances are you've been on a diet of some sort at some time in your life. Men are more inclined to wait until they've got middle-age spread or a pot belly before they make an effort to cut down on fried breakfasts or go without the odd pint or two.

But apart from your appearance, and the way you feel about yourself, how over-weight are you as far as your health is concerned?

The chart below gives you the answer – and you may be surprised to find that, in health terms anyway, you're allowed to be a little fuller in the figure than current fashion dictates.

Check your weight here

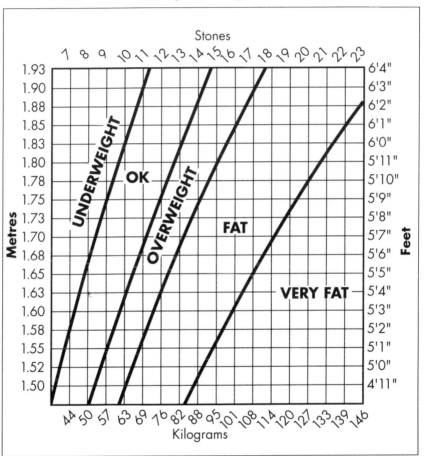

Weigh yourself without clothes, and measure your height without shoes. Then check yourself against the chart: run your finger up from your weight to a point level with your height, and read off which band you're in.

Underweight

Are you eating enough? You probably need to eat more of the healthy balance of foods outlined in this chapter. If dieting is ruling your life, or you're hooked on laxatives or slimming pills, or you deliberately bring food back up after meals, you have an eating disorder which may need medical attention.

OK

Congratulations – you're in the optimum weight range for your health. But you may still be eating an unhealthy balance of foods in other respects – particularly in terms of saturated fats and fibre. Follow the guidelines later in this chapter.

Overweight

You need to lose some weight – but there's no need to rush at it. No crash dieting please – it's not at all a healthy way to slim. The way to tackle this moderate degree of plumpness is not to 'diet', but to change to a more healthy and natural balance of everyday eating, and build up your physical activity a little – in other words, be more of a 'hunter-gatherer'. In this way, you'll lose weight steadily, at the rate of about 0.5kg (1lb) a week – which sounds dreadfully slow, but is actually about 6kg (nearly a stone) in just three months. And because you change your way of eating, the weight will stay off.

Fat

You have a real weight problem, and it's likely to affect your health if you don't get any slimmer. The most effective way to shed this extra body fat is to lose it slowly – no more than 1kg (2lb) a week. This means changing the way you eat following the simple principles outlined in this chapter. Aim to consume about 500-750 fewer calories a day than you do at the moment. Not a huge sacrifice – but it should be enough to send your weight in a downward direction.

Very fat

You are seriously obese and urgently need to lose weight because it's almost certainly damaging your health. No doubt you're only too well aware of this, and have already sought the advice of your doctor. But if not, you really need to do so – sooner rather than later. In the mean time, use the principles outlined in this chapter to lose no more than 1kg (2lb) a week by consuming up to 750 fewer calories a day than you do at present.

Everybody's different

Averages are all very well, but what makes life interesting is that everybody's different. We all inherit different body shapes, different metabolisms, different rates of ageing. And we have different lifestyles, with different eating and drinking habits, taking different amounts of exercise, coping with different degrees of stress, and indulging in different vices.

All these factors affect our nutritional balance and in particular our need for calories. It's one of life's fundamental injustices that some people can stuff themselves silly with all manner of fatty and sugary excesses without gaining an ounce, whilst others have only to peep at a profiterole and they pile on pounds.

Over the past few years, scientists have begun to unravel the mystery of how our bodies differ so widely in the way they cope with extra calories.

One basic difference is our sex. Normal-weight women have about fifty per cent more body fat than normal-weight men. That's thanks to evolution again. The extra fat not only gives women their characteristic curves but also provides them with a reserve energy supply that could, in times of famine, keep them alive and able to suckle their young. Men tend to be leaner and more muscular, which, in evolutionary terms, made them better hunters and defenders. Muscle burns up more calories than fatty tissue does, even when it's doing nothing. So, not only do active men burn up more calories than equally active women, but the same is also true of idle men and equally idle women. It isn't fair is it?

This is tied to another way in which we all differ from each other – the 'tickover' of our metabolism – our basal metabolic rate (BMR). This determines how fast we burn up calories when we're just doing nothing – in other words, the calories needed just to run our various bodily systems and processes whilst we're at rest. Yes, even thinking burns up calories.

People with low basal metabolic rates tend to put on fat more easily. Starvation lowers the BMR. There is some evidence to suggest that it may be possible to increase the BMR by exercising regularly. Some people have metabolisms that respond to daily vigorous aerobic exercise (such as brisk walking, running or swimming) by speeding up, not just during exercise, but for quite a while after it. Just think – if you're one of these fortunate souls -providing you exercise enough during the day, you can actually slim whilst you sleep!

Another factor is the body's central heating system, called thermogenesis. This is a mechanism for dissipating excess calories in the form of heat. Naturally lean people are better at it than fat people – which explains their difference in weight. If a naturally thin person is fed a high-fat meal, the body responds by generating more heat – rather like switching on an extra bar of their internal electric fire. But a person who is prone to overweight, even though he or she may be slim at the time, will respond to the meal by straightaway laying down fat. Unfortunately, this thermogenic effect tends to diminish with age – which explains why even naturally slim people tend to get plumper as they get older.

Apples and pears

Not only are women naturally plumper than men, but the extra adipose tissue tends to be in different places (thank goodness!). Women put the inches on mostly around the hips and thighs, and perhaps the breasts and shoulders. For men, it's mostly around the waist and chin. Men are 'apples', women 'pears'.

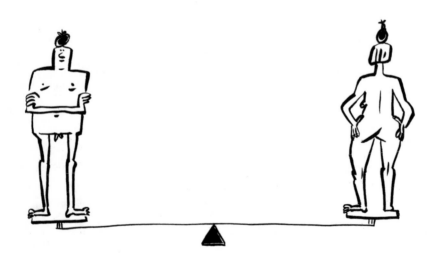

Men tend to be 'apples' – women 'pears'

These different body shapes carry different health risks. Studies have shown that the 'apple' form of obesity is more worrying from the health point of view than the 'pear' form. It's more likely to lead to high blood pressure, diabetes and heart disease – even after correcting for other factors such as gender itself. It also supports the view that the pear-shape is biologically normal and natural for women, and helps to explain why fat around the hips and thighs, sometimes called 'cellulite', is the hardest to shift.

Is cellulite special?

Yes, in the sense that it's meant to be there. It's fat, just like any other body fat, but it's more under the control of the female hormones than ordinary fat elsewhere in the body. It's the main last-ditch store of energy in times of famine. Although, along with other body fat, it can be reduced by dieting, it's the most resistant to change. The fat cells in cellulite hang on to their precious contents long after other fat cells have given up. Many women are as skinny as a rake from the waist up, but full in their hips and thighs – much to their chagrin.

Unfortunately, there's no easy answer to this – no special creams or potions to 'dissolve' the cellulite or break down the fat-forming tissue; no special diet that targets hips and thighs; no exercises to remove the fat selectively from the offending areas. You just have to stay as slim as is sensible, by following the healthy eating guidelines in this chapter.

Pacing yourself

The crucial thing about the healthy eating approach to successful slimming is to take it slowly and steadily. Your metabolism is smarter than you think – it adapts itself to the calorific content of your diet and makes adjustments to conserve energy. If you go on a crash diet, your body chemistry recognises the threat of imminent starvation and shuts down a lot of energy-consuming processes in order to conserve fuel. It adopts a sort of 'siege economy' and instead of burning up lots of calories it stores more of them as body fat.

This is why so many people reach a depressing 'plateau' with their weight loss. They do well to start with – perhaps shedding a stone or two without much difficulty – and then nothing. The scales refuse to drop any lower. What has happened is that their metabolism has readjusted to the sudden very low calorie intake, and found a new equilibrium.

Cracking the plateau

The way to avoid this is to lose weight much more slowly, so that you don't trigger the 'siege' reaction. You fool your metabolism into thinking that everything's quite normal, and it doesn't need to readjust any of its settings. You can also step up your exercise, so that your metabolism is forced to burn calories – it has no choice.

Yo-yo dieting

Don't be fooled by diets that promise you that you'll lose a lot of weight very quickly. Unfortunately, it's the wrong sort of weight. That first half-stone (3kg) or so is virtually all water – yes, water. This is because the first energy stores your body turns to if it's being starved are the deposits of quick-release glycogen in your muscles and liver. And when glycogen is broken down it produces water along with the energy. Once the glycogen is gone, you hit your first big plateau. You get despondent, you give up the diet, and you put all the weight back on again – the all-too-familiar 'yo-yo' dieting fiasco. Again, taking it slowly will avoid this problem because you give your body enough time to break down body fat rather than the quick-release glycogen.

Will-power

A staggering ninety-five per cent of dieters fail because they try to lose too much weight too quickly. They either give up the struggle halfway through, or put the weight straight back on as soon as they stop dieting.

The will-power you need to lose weight successfully is not so much the will-power to fight the temptation to scoff a chocolate bar or a cream cake – although that can be tough enough – but the will-power to help you fight the temptation to go on a crash diet. Strict, rigid, regimented diets may make you feel you're doing something definite and positive – it's easier to obey strict rules about exactly what you can eat, and exactly when. But this only works up to a point – and then all-too-often it collapses. The reason why it collapses is that 'dieting' isn't natural and it isn't part of normal healthy living.

The answer is to harness your will-power to change to a healthier balance of eating in which the key nutrients are in balance with each other, and the calorie content is in balance with the energy requirements of your lifestyle. Follow the basic guidelines in this chapter. That way, the weight you lose will stay lost and the benefits of being slimmer will be lasting.

And don't rush at it. Give yourself time. If you want to look lithe and lissome on the beach, start changing your eating habits at least three months, and preferably six months, beforehand. Better still, start now for the holiday after next – and for the rest of your life.

The classic dieter's mistake

Don't be tempted to weigh yourself too often. Once a week is quite often enough – at about the same time of day. The classic dieter's mistake is to keep checking their weight every day – in some sad cases, two or three times a day. This is mental torture, because one's weight naturally fluctuates perhaps two or three pounds (about a kilogram) during twenty-four hours, depending on how full your bladder and bowels are, when you last ate or drank, and even whether you've been standing up or lying down.

Women should expect to be a little heavier in the days before each period, when their premenstrual hormones cause fluid retention.

Mark your present weight on the chart below with a cross on the left-hand scale, and put today's date (or whenever you want to start) at the left-hand end of the timescale along the bottom. Assuming a weight loss rate of about 0.5kg (1lb) a week, mark another cross 6kg (about 1 stone) lighter in 3 months' time, and another 12kg (nearly 2 stone) lighter in 6 months' time. Join the two crosses with a line. Now do the same thing assuming a weight loss rate of 1kg (2lb) a week, and draw another line.

Weigh yourself just once a week, at about the same time of day, and enter your weight on the chart. You should aim to keep your weekly progress between the two lines.

Weight loss progress chart

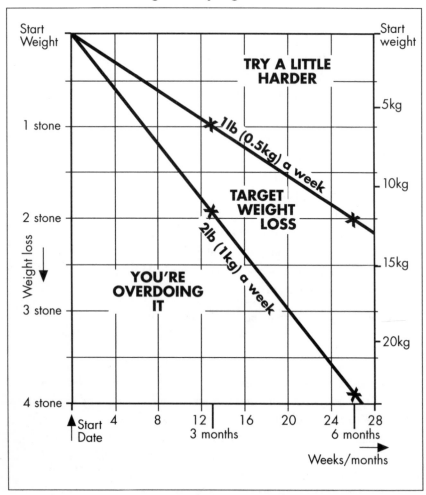

Where are the calories?

It may come as a surprise to some people to learn that such well-known fillers as bread, potatoes, pasta, rice and other starchy staples are not particularly fattening. Indeed, this is precisely because they fill your tummy with satisfying, low-calorie bulk. Instead, the slimmer's real enemies are high-fat or high-sugar foods, densely packed with calories – and also that enticing calorie-rich fluid, alcohol. Fat, in particular, has twice as many calories as the same weight of starchy food.

Sugar gives you virtually nothing but 'empty calories' – no vitamins, no minerals, no protein. Don't make the mistake of thinking that sugar gives you instant energy and will act as a pick-you-up. This is a misunderstanding of the word 'energy'. The only instant energy sugar gives is calories – neat calories. Any uplifting effect on your mood or banishing of fatigue is mostly psychological. It probably harks back to the days of your childhood when sweets were a treat.

FATS AND THE HEART

If you were to drop in on your GP, you might find yourself having a conversation about the health of your parents, your immediate family and any serious heart or blood pressure problems which may have affected them. When the GP gets round to you, it will be to ask about your occupation, lifestyle and diet. In particular, how much fat you eat, tobacco you smoke and alcohol you drink.

By putting your family history together with your present lifestyle, your GP is attempting to assess your risk of coronary heart disease. You may be asked for a blood test to look at the amount of cholesterol and other fats (lipids) you have in your bloodstream.

On its own, a high cholesterol level is not necessarily significant – only when linked to a strong family history of heart disease, high blood pressure or cigarette smoking does it become more important. Some families have a genetic tendency to produce more cholesterol, and they have a higher risk of heart disease. If you have such a family history you should certainly have your cholesterol levels checked and reduce your intake of fats. Even without any family history of heart disease or high levels of cholesterol, it makes sense to reduce the amount of fat you eat.

Furring up

Any hard-working muscle has to have plenty of oxygen to fire its energy system, and a rapid means of removing spent fuel. The crucial requirement is a rich blood supply to do both jobs. This is why all muscles are so red – they have a very dense network of blood vessels.

Heart, showing coronary arteries

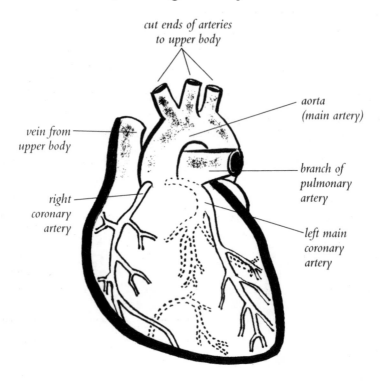

cut ends of arteries
to upper body

aorta
(main artery)

vein from
upper body

branch of
pulmonary
artery

right
coronary
artery

left main
coronary
artery

How a coronary artery can become clogged

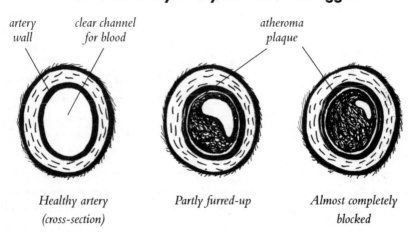

artery
wall

clear channel
for blood

atheroma
plaque

Healthy artery
(cross-section)

Partly furred-up

Almost completely
blocked

No muscle has a greater need for a thoroughly effective blood supply than the heart muscle itself. To ensure this, it receives freshly oxygenated blood through its own private arteries – the coronary arteries – which are the very first branches off the aorta, the main artery leaving the heart.

The coronary arteries are only about as wide as a drinking straw and encircle the top of the heart (corona is Latin for 'crown') before branching into smaller vessels that course all over its surface and plunge deep into its muscle, branching again and again until every part of the heart is reached.

Because the heart has to cope with such varying demands – working up to twenty times as hard when you're exercising as when you're at rest – the coronary arteries are able to become much wider in order to carry any extra blood needed. Young people's coronary arteries can do this much more effectively than older people's. In middle age, the arterial walls begin to stiffen and lose their elasticity (like so many other parts of the body!). This can have important consequences if the arteries also happen to be 'furring up' inside with fatty deposits.

If a coronary artery, or major branch, becomes so narrow or clogged that part of the heart is deprived of an adequate blood supply, the person will feel the characteristic heavy cardiac pain in their chest, jaw or shoulders. This usually first becomes apparent during heavy exertion, or at times of excitement or emotion, when the heart is beating faster or needs more oxygen. These are classic times for angina to strike.

If a clot, or thrombus, forms in a furred-up coronary artery, or its branch, it can very rapidly constrict the blood flow still more, bringing on worsening angina – 'crescendo angina' – unrelieved by rest.

If the clot builds up so rapidly that it completely blocks the artery (coronary thrombosis), the part of the heart muscle supplied by that blood vessel is suddenly deprived of all its sustenance. This causes the classic pain and other symptoms of a heart attack – the biggest killer in the Western world.

Fatty deposits

The fatty deposits that cause all this furring-up are called atheromatous plaques. They are whitish, stiff, ragged patches consisting mainly of cholesterol and calcium. They begin as little more than microscopic fatty streaks in one's teenage years or twenties. But they very gradually thicken up, slowly clogging the arteries. This build-up is much faster in some people than others. It partly depends on family history, partly on blood pressure, and partly on the level of cholesterol in the bloodstream, which in turn is affected by the amount of fat in the diet, especially saturated fat.

What exactly is cholesterol?

It's a soft, waxy, fat-like substance, with the consistency of warm candle grease, which plays a vital part in every cell of the body. It's a key component of cell membranes, helping to regulate what goes in and out of the cell. It's an important component of bile, the digestive fluid used to help break down fats. It's used in the body's manufacture of natural steroids, including certain sex hormones. And it helps to keep our arteries leak-proof.

So we need cholesterol. But problems arise if we have too much in our bloodstream. The higher the level, the faster the furring-up with atheromatous deposits, and the greater the risk of angina, heart attack, and other disorders caused by clogged arteries, such as strokes.

Where does it come from?

Surprisingly, at least two-thirds of the body's cholesterol is manufactured in our own liver, by converting fat, especially saturated fat. Most of the rest is synthesised by cells in the small intestine, again from fat. Only a very minor proportion comes from cholesterol already present in our food. Much more important is the amount of fat, especially saturated fat, that we eat.

Saturated fats

Technically speaking, these are fats or oils that are high in saturated fatty acids, but in practical terms they're the fats found mainly in foods of animal origin – meat and meat products, milk, butter, cheese and other dairy produce – and also in some plant oils, most notably palm oil, coconut oil and 'hardened' (hydrogenated) vegetable oils.

Unsaturated fats

These come in two types – polyunsaturated and monounsaturated.

The polys are better known and, broadly speaking, are 'good' fats as far as the heart is concerned. The richest sources of polys are from plant-seeds and fish – most notably sunflower oil, safflower oil, soya oil, corn oil and fish oils. The polys in these oils not only have an anti-atheroma effect, but also seem to render the blood less liable to thrombosis.

Many fats and oils of both plant and animal origin are high in monounsaturates. The richest sources are olive, peanut (groundnut) and rapeseed oil. Monounsaturates are also thought to have some anti-atheroma effect. Needless to say, for your heart's sake, both monos and polys should be used to replace saturated fats whenever possible. One of the great benefits of the Mediterranean diet is thought to be its reliance on olive oil and fish.

What do Inuits and the Japanese have in common? Well, they both eat lots of fish and both have very low rates of heart disease. What's more, the lowest rates in Japan are among the people of Okinawa, whose fish consumption is about twice that of mainland Japanese.

In a twenty-year study, Dutch researchers have found a clear relationship between the amount of fish eaten and the risk of coronary heart disease – the more fish, the fewer heart attacks. The most important fish for your heart are those with darker, more oily flesh – sardines, tuna, mackerel, herring, pilchards and salmon. These are rich sources of long-chain polyunsaturated fats, which have a clot-reducing and anti-clogging effect on your coronary arteries. So, fish is good for your heart as well as your brains.

But, remember the calories

We mustn't let the notion of 'good fats' and 'bad fats' allow us to forget that all fats and oils (oils are simply fats that are liquid at room temperature) are packed with calories, absolutely chock full of them. Oils have just as many as hard fats. Soft margarines just as many as butter or lard. So, if you're going to eat more oily fish, or cook with sunflower or olive oil, it's important to cut down on calories from elsewhere, especially by eating much less saturated fat.

Where's the fat?

Always check labels carefully so that you know how much saturated and unsat-

Main sources of fat in the typical household diet

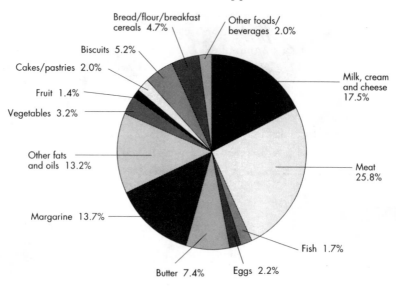

Bread/flour/breakfast cereals 4.7%

Other foods/beverages 2.0%

Biscuits 5.2%

Cakes/pastries 2.0%

Fruit 1.4%

Vegetables 3.2%

Other fats and oils 13.2%

Margarine 13.7%

Butter 7.4%

Eggs 2.2%

Fish 1.7%

Meat 25.8%

Milk, cream and cheese 17.5%

Main sources of saturated fatty acids in the typical household diet

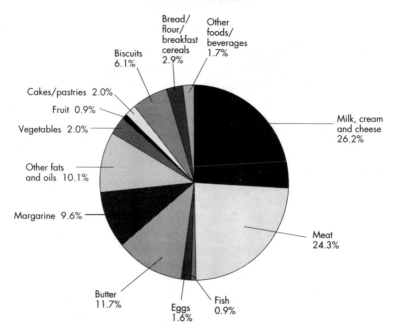

Bread/flour/breakfast cereals 2.9%

Other foods/beverages 1.7%

Biscuits 6.1%

Cakes/pastries 2.0%

Fruit 0.9%

Vegetables 2.0%

Other fats and oils 10.1%

Margarine 9.6%

Butter 11.7%

Eggs 1.6%

Fish 0.9%

Meat 24.3%

Milk, cream and cheese 26.2%

urated fat there is in the food you're buying. Remember that most of the fat in our diet is saturated and comes from meat and dairy products. Look for lower fat alternatives – leaner cuts of meat, chicken, white fish, low-fat sausages, semi-skimmed or skimmed milk, low-fat spreads, low-fat cheeses, low-fat dressings and sauces. Beware also the 'hidden fats' in things like chocolate, biscuits, cakes and pastries.

When you prepare food, cut the visible fat off meat, grill rather than fry, and skim the excess fat off casseroles.

FIBRE AND DIGESTION

Roughen up

Just about the biggest change in nutritional thinking over the past couple of decades has been the realisation that what we used to dismiss as mere 'roughage' is actually a very important part of our diet. Now with the more dignified name 'dietary fibre' it's one of the main food components of which most of us aren't getting enough.

Fibre

The very word conjures up images of sackcloth and ashes, or cardboard, self-denial and punishment. But how wrong, how very wrong.

Fibre comes from plants – the cell walls of fruits, vegetables, grains, shoots, leaves and nuts. The greengrocer's shop or stall is a riot of colourful, vibrant, delectable treats of flavoursome fibre. There's lots in the baker's too. And on the supermarket shelves amongst the rice and pasta, the lentils and beans, the fruit and vegetables.

Smoothage

The fibre in these foods acts as a gift-wrap for the vitamins, minerals, proteins and starch that our body needs in abundance. These goodies are released by chewing and by enzymes in our digestive system before they are absorbed into the bloodstream. The fibre itself is not digested or absorbed, but is important in providing the colon (large intestine) with soft bulk to ease the passage of other food residue through to the bowel. In this sense, it's acting more as 'smoothage' than roughage.

This smoothing, bulking action is crucial for the health of our colon. It helps to prevent constipation, and reduces pressures in the colon keeping the bowel contents shifting along nicely. This in turn protects us from various ills.

Studies around the world have pointed to a link between our modern refined low-fibre diet and several common diseases of the developed world – piles, diverticular disease, varicose veins, appendicitis, diabetes and bowel cancer. All are comparatively rare in countries where the diet is high in fibre-rich starchy staples like rice, sago and cassava.

In rural Africa, for example, the average time taken for food to pass through the digestive system is about thirty-six hours. In Britain it varies from about three days in young people to as long as two weeks in the elderly. Rural Africans eat four or five times as much fibre as people in the UK. Vegetarians in Britain eat about twice as much fibre as the national average, and are much less likely to suffer from the diseases mentioned above.

Proportion of fibre in selected foods

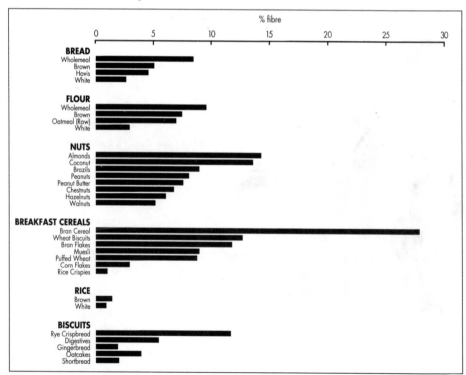

Proportion of fibre in selected foods *continued*

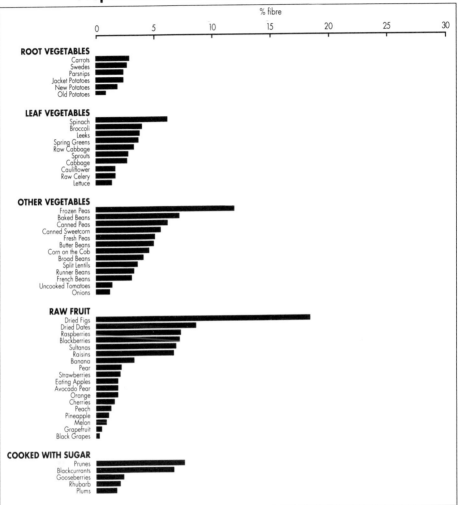

Let loose

About four out of ten people in this country admit to being constipated, and about one in five takes laxatives: millions of pounds' worth every year. What a waste.

The best and most natural way to get things moving is to eat more fibre-rich foods – more wholegrain cereals, wholemeal bread, potatoes, rice, pasta, pulses (beans and peas), vegetables, fruit and nuts. Feast on all these wonderful things.

21

Fibre-wrapped goodies

Because they are relatively low in calories and high in vitamins and minerals, fibre-rich starchy staples such as potatoes, rice, pasta, cereals or bread, should form the basis of each meal. The World Health Organisation recommends that at least half our calories should come from these complex carbohydrate foods. That's about twice as much as the average person eats at present.

The WHO also says we should each eat at least 400 grams (about 1 lb) of fruit, salads and vegetables (not including potatoes) a day. Tinned, frozen or fresh – they all count. This means eating about five portions of these good things each and every day.

VITAMINS AND MINERALS

Panacea or put-on?

Leaf through almost any of the women's magazines, or health and fitness glossies, and you'll find page after page of articles or adverts extolling the virtues of multi-vitamin supplements. It's very big business indeed. The advertisers go on about the stresses and strains of modern living, rushed meals, junk snacks and inadequate slimming diets. Some of them claim that their particular vitamin cocktail can even improve your IQ.

But the truth is that most people really don't need to take extra vitamins or minerals. By following the simple healthy eating guidelines in this chapter, you can get all the 'vits and mins' your body needs – with plenty to spare: Vitamin C from all those extra fruits and vegetables, iron from lean meat and leafy greens, calcium from low-fat dairy products, and so on.

To make sure that the foods you eat are as nutritious as possible, it's important that they are either eaten fresh, cooked lightly or stored properly so that they don't lose their nutrient value. Vitamin C and the B vitamins, for example, are easily destroyed by poor storage or over-cooking.

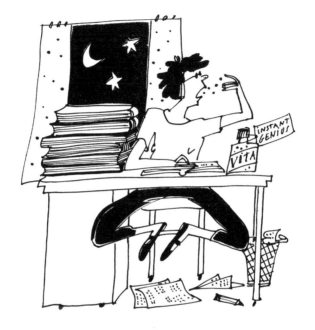

Unfortunately, extra vitamins don't make young people extra intelligent

Frozen, chilled, dried or packaged foods can be as good a source of vitamins and minerals as 'fresh' foods. Frozen peas, for example, are easy to store, easy to cook, and highly nutritious, retaining their nutrients so well that they have more vitamins than fresh peas that have been sitting around too long.

Try to avoid over-cooking vegetables, otherwise most of the vitamins end up in the cooking water. So, cook for only a short time in as little water as possible. Better still, use a steamer or microwave, or stir-fry in a very little oil.

Who needs supplements?

Although most of us will get more than enough vitamins and minerals by eating a varied and balanced diet, there are some people who may need to take supplements. For instance, extra iron may be needed for women with heavy periods. Women who are planning to become pregnant should take folic acid tablets until they are twelve weeks into the pregnancy. Some Asian children may need extra Vitamin D to help prevent rickets caused by a lack of sunlight on their skin. Elderly men living alone are notorious for their poor diet and may well need to take a multi-vitamin and mineral supplement. The same applies to many people whose appetite is poor, or who are recovering from illness or an operation.

Mega dangers

For most people, taking extra vitamins and minerals will not be extra good for them. On the contrary, there are potential dangers in having some of the mega-doses on offer. Vitamin A, for example, is very toxic in large doses. There are also concerns that megadoses of Vitamin C might lead to kidney stones. With some large vitamin intakes, the body may have problems adjusting when the supplement is stopped, and there is a worry that certain excess minerals can interfere with the action of others. Last but not least, a steady supply of vitamin supplements can seriously damage your family budget.

ACE high

There's increasing evidence that certain plant foods, particularly green and yellow vegetables, berries and citrus fruits, help to confer some protection against the development of cancers. These anti-cancer effects are thought to be thanks to the Vitamins C, E and beta-carotene (Vitamin A) which act as anti-oxidants, neutralising so-called 'free radicals' – by-products of cell activity in every tissue of the body. Excess of free radicals is highly damaging and has been linked not only to the triggering of cancers but also atheroma deposits and heart disease.

Traditional national diets rich in Vitamins A, C and E - the ACE vitamins - are associated with lower rates of cancer and heart disease. The Mediterranean diet, with its abundance of fresh fruit, salads and lightly cooked vegetables is a classic example.

Main sources of Vitamins A, C and E

Vitamin A
Carrots
Cheese
Dried apricots
Eggs
Green leafy vegetables
Liver
Tomatoes

Vitamin C
Blackcurrants
Cirtus fruits
Green vegetables
Potatoes
Tomatoes

Vitamin E
Cereals
Eggs
Vegetable oil

THE RIGHT BALANCE

For modern developed nations such as ours, diseases related to deficiencies in the diet, such as scurvy and rickets, are thankfully rare. For millions in the developing World, they are a very real and constant threat. Children with beri-beri, kwashi-orkor (bloated bodies with little resistance to infection caused by protein deficiency) and rickets are still common sights on our television screens as successive famines are reported from various parts of the world.

Paradoxically, we also watch television dramas highlighting the damage done by our affluent diet – no hospital soap would be complete without the heart attack victim. Our dietary diseases are caused by a surfeit rather than shortage. The developed world is plagued by diseases of affluence – heart disease, cancers, diabetes, strokes, dental decay – the result of too much fatty, sugary and salty food, and not enough simple fibre-rich starchy staples.

Clear guidelines

Experts throughout the world have come to the conclusion that the average diet of developed nations is far too high in saturated fat from meat, meat products and dairy foods, and far too low in fruit, vegetables and fibre-rich starchy foods such as bread, cereals and potatoes.

The World Health Organisation has outlined the following recommendations:

- **Eat much more fruit, vegetables and salads.**
  The WHO recommends a minimum of 400g (just under 1lb) a day, not counting potatoes. It means eating at least five portions of fruit and vegetables (including beans) a day.

- **Eat much more bread, potatoes, cereals, rice, lentils or other starchy food.**
  The WHO recommends that starchy foods (complex carbohydrates) should provide 50–70 per cent of our calories. That's about twice as much as they do at present on average. It means we should double our intake of these and other fibre-rich starchy foods.

- **Think carefully about meat, meat products, full-fat dairy products, eggs, cooking oils and other fatty foods.**
  The main problem here is fat, especially saturated fat. The WHO recommends that we derive no more than 30 per cent of our energy (calories) from fats and oils of all types, and preferably less than that (but not less than 15 per cent for fear of missing out on essential fatty acids and fat-soluble vitamins). This means that most of us should cut our fat intake by between one-third and one-half, especially from foods high in saturated fat.

- **Consider chicken, turkey and fish as alternatives.**
  Poultry meat has less saturated fat than most red meat. Oily fish are fatty, but relatively low in saturated fats and high in beneficial polyunsaturates. White fish contain very little fat of any kind.

- **Eat sugary foods much less often.**
  Refined sugar is a concentrated form of calories but has no other nutrient value. Eating and drinking fewer sugary things will help you control your weight and keep tooth decay and gum disease at bay. The WHO says we have no need whatsoever for refined sugar, and

recommends that no more than 10 per cent of our calories should come from this source. For the average person, this means cutting sugar in all its various guises in our diet by up to half.

- **Cut down on salt.**

  The sodium in salt is essential – but we eat far too much of it. It's tasty and it's cheap, so manufacturers load it into all sorts of products. A high-salt diet is thought to be an important cause of high blood pressure and stroke. The salt in bread, along with that naturally occurring in various foods, is quite enough for our needs. We should avoid salty foods, and add less salt in the kitchen and at the table. The WHO recommends that our current intake should be at least halved.

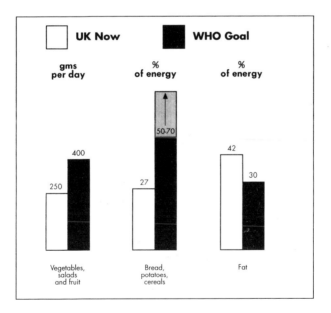

Too boring, too fiddly, too expensive?

Some of the most enticing and delicious cuisines in the world are also among the healthiest: traditional Mediterranean food, for instance, with its emphasis on fresh, lightly cooked vegetables, or salads, together with bread, pasta or rice, abundant fish and a little meat, topped with aromatic herbs and rounded off with the freshest of fruits. So too is the food of the Indian subcontinent, largely based on rice and vegetables, with its amazing range of exotic and scintillating spices, or Oriental food, again rice-based or with oodles of noodles plus lots of fresh vegetables – stir-fried very quickly to preserve vitamins – with chicken, duck or, certainly in Japan, fish galore.

Nor need healthy eating be fiddly. Reaching for an apple, or opening a carton of low-fat yoghurt, isn't too troublesome. Cutting a thick slice of wholemeal bread, or heating some baked beans, needn't take too much effort. A healthy salad can be thrown together in a trice. Steaming fish or leafy vegetables takes not much longer. And if you have a freezer and microwave, you can make your own 'convenience' foods for the whole week at one go.

A healthy diet needn't break your budget. Steak is expensive, but chicken isn't. Salmon's a luxury, but tuna's good value. Vegetables and fruit in season are real bargains, especially from the market. Frozen foods are not much more expensive than fresh, but always available, with less waste, and are usually just as nutritious as fresh foods because the vitamins are well preserved. Staples like wholemeal bread, potatoes, cereals, wholegrain rice, yams and cassava are all relatively cheap. On the other hand, take-aways and pre-cooked microwave dinners are quite pricey – and, if you have them often, can really push your food bill through the roof.

EATING WELL

So much for the theory – but there's little fun just reading about delicious food; the proof, as they say, is in the eating. Here's how to go about it.

Your shopping basket

Armed with the basic principles outlined above, it's time to fill up the shopping basket, or trolley, with some healthier alternatives.

Fruit and vegetables:
Linger for a long time in the greengrocer section of your supermarket, or a shop or market stall. Here you could fill your whole basket with luscious delights. Choose a selection of fresh fruit (including lemons), plus potatoes, greens, carrots, onions, and salad vegetables – whatever takes your fancy. Move on and stock up with frozen vegetables too – peas, beans, broccoli. At

the tinned section buy baked beans, sweetcorn, chick peas, r
beans, tomatoes. Look for vegetables without added salt, and fru.
natural juice. Choose unsweetened fruit juices.

Dairy foods, fats and oils, cooked meats:
Choose semi-skimmed or skimmed milk (but whole milk for under-fives).
Low-fat plain or fruit yoghurts and fromage frais. Lower-fat cheeses.
Polyunsaturated margarine and low-fat spread (one for cooking, the other
for spreading). Eggs to be used sparingly. Sunflower, corn or olive oil. Lean
ham. Low-fat sausages.

Fresh and frozen meat:
Lean cuts, lean mince. Chicken or chicken pieces, turkey thighs. Low-fat
burgers. Or try vegetarian alternatives.

Fresh, frozen or tinned fish:
Any fish, white or oily. Steady with the roes (high in cholesterol). The same
goes for shellfish. Frozen fish (yes, even fish fingers). Tinned tuna, sardines
pilchards, salmon. Anchovies for seasoning only (extremely salty).

The balance of good health

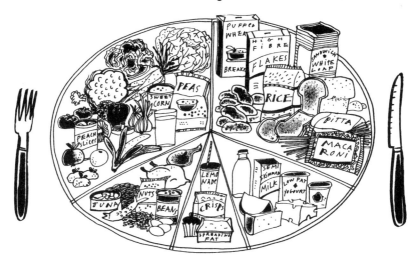

Other foods:
Wholemeal flour for breadmaking and pastries. Baker's yeast. Cornflour or arrowroot for thickening. Rolled oats and oatbran, nuts and dried fruit for muesli. Wholegrain breakfast cereals. Brown rice. Wholewheat pasta. Wholemeal bread, rolls, pitta. Wholegrain crispbread. Dried pulses – beans, peas and lentils. Herbs and spices.

You can get all these things in your local supermarket – as long as you read the labels carefully. But why not shop around a little? Try the specialist shops in the high street. Talk to the shopkeepers and gain from their knowledge. For keener prices, there's the street market. And don't forget your local wholefood store for a wider selection of dried pulses, grains, nuts, fruits and pasta.

Healthier cooking

This isn't a cookbook, so there's only room to make a few key points, but here are the essentials:

- Whenever possible, eat fruit or vegetables raw or only lightly cooked – preferably steamed. Wash thoroughly to remove pesticide residues.
- Grill or bake rather than fry. Bake with foil to retain the flavour.
- If you need to fry, use unsaturated oil (such as sunflower, corn or olive oil), or dry-fry in a coated pan. Stir-frying in a wok is an excellent and fast way to cook small chunks of meat, fish, shellfish and vegetables.
- If the children insist on chips, use oven-ready, or deep-fry by cutting chips thickly and putting into very hot fat (but not so hot that it smokes – fire!).
- Roast meat on a rack over the roasting tin so that the fat is separated and can be poured off. Use a little polyunsaturated oil for basting vegetables.
- Casseroles and pot-roasts. Skim off the fat that rises to the surface or cook the dish the day before and lift off the hardened layer of fat before reheating.
- Boiling, poaching and steaming. Good low-fat ways of cooking – but use a minimum of water for a minimum of time to preserve vulnerable vitamins. Poaching or steaming is best for fish, especially white fish. Steaming leafy vegetables preserves their colour, flavour and crunchiness.
- Microwave cooking is fast enough to preserve much of the nutrient content and flavour. Particularly good for potatoes, vegetables and fruit. A jacket potato takes just four minutes.

Snacks and treats

Life isn't worth living without snacks and treats – especially for children of all ages. Some of the healthiest nibbles are also the nicest – apples, pears, tangerines, bananas and unsalted nuts, not to forget crunchy salad things like celery, carrots, cherry tomatoes and peppers. Dried fruit, raisins and dates are good, and not too sweet. Low-sugar muesli or wholegrain cereal with semi-skimmed milk is a filling snack at any time of day.

And if you really crave a cream-filled doughnut or a chocolate biscuit … well, go on, have it. But just the one, mind! Only a little of what you fancy does you good!

KEEP MOVING

MOVE IT

Who, me?

We all know the health benefits of active living. We've heard them scores of times – at school, on TV and the radio. We've skimmed the articles in magazines and newspapers. We've got the picture.

We know that being more active helps us to keep in shape and cope better with life's stresses and strains, that it can help us feel good about ourselves, and more relaxed about life.

What for?

We know that regular activity builds up and maintains our strength, suppleness and staying power, that it keeps our bones and joints strong, and helps to protect our heart.

And we know that leisure activities are a great way of meeting people, making friends and having fun.

So, why, despite the boom in active pursuits and leisure centres, are four out of five people still far too inactive for their own good? Why do most people still regard exercise as something others are welcome to indulge in, but which they themselves would rather avoid if at all possible?

Excuses, excuses

Perhaps it's because it's all too easy to come up with excuses for taking the easy way out. Here are a few of the classic lines that you may well find yourself coming up with – and the counter-arguments for making a bit more effort.

Excuses

I haven't got the time. I'm far too busy

This is a favourite one. A sort of don't-bother-me-with-trifles now excuse. It sounds reasonable enough – but it's based on the false idea that to be more active you have to carve great chunks out of your routine. Not so. There are all sorts of ways you can fit active alternatives into your everyday life. Walking up stairs instead of taking the lift, for instance. Getting off the bus a stop or two earlier. Walking or cycling to the shops or station instead of taking the car. Playing more active games with the kids. Taking the dog for a jog. And even more dedicated activity sessions, like swimming, badminton or dancing, needn't take up too much time – once or twice a week can make a big difference.

It's too much like hard work

Who said anything about hard work? You've just got to do a little more than you're used to, that's all. Anyway, it won't seem at all like hard work if you choose activities you enjoy and build up slowly and gradually.

As you get better at it you'll enjoy it even more and you won't want to give it up. What's more, you'll find that active living doesn't tire you – it energises you.

I'm not the sporty type

Come on. You don't have to do 'sporty' things to be more active. You don't need lots of special gear to go walking in the park or country. You don't need to get involved in team games if you don't want to.

Forget all those memories of PE at school if they're painful for you. Just find ways of moving about a bit more, and enjoying yourself while you're at it.

What I need is relaxation

Well, believe it or not, exercise can be just the thing to help you unwind and relax. It relieves stress by taking your mind off your problems. After vigorous activity, you'll feel warm, comfortable and tension-free. It can greatly improve the quality of your sleep. And recent studies have shown that exercise can also lift depression.

I've got young children to look after

That's a pretty active lifestyle in itself – all that lifting and carrying and bending and stretching – but, with a bit of organising, you can also do active things you enjoy. Some sports and leisure centres have childcare facilities at reasonable prices. Or you could get together with a group of other people with young children and share the babysitting.

If you have to stay at home, why not put on an exercise tape and let the young ones join in? They'll love it.

I'm too fat, too old, too out of condition, etc.

Then you're just the sort of person who has most to gain from being more active. It will burn up excess calories, reset your metabolic thermostat and help to crack the plateau you may be stuck with in your slimming programme.

It's never too late to use your body a little more, and become a little fitter. Whatever your age or state of decrepitude, you can find some activity that suits you. If you're worried about your heart, or breathing, or joints, or any other medical condition, have a word with your doctor. But, broadly speaking, the less fit you are to start with, the sooner you'll notice the benefits.

Simply being more supple and mobile will decrease the risk of injury from falling – one of the main causes of broken hips in elderly people.

A more active lifestyle will improve your mental outlook, help fight illness and encourage you to meet people, whatever your age or medical condition.

WHY BOTHER?

Active living: plus points for women

1. Strengthens bones, which helps to prevent osteoporosis and to avoid fractures in later life.

2. Prepares the body for the extra demands of pregnancy and childbirth by toning the system and strengthening the heart. Also tones body and strengthens heart even if not pregnant!

3. Helps you get back into shape after a baby by tightening ligaments, toning up flabby muscles, and shedding excess weight.

4. Tones the abdominal and pelvic muscles preventing stress incontinence.

5. Gets you out of the workplace, be it office, factory or home.

6. Gives you time to yourself, free from the demands of work, children or partners.

7. Improves your stamina, ability to cope, sex life and self-esteem.

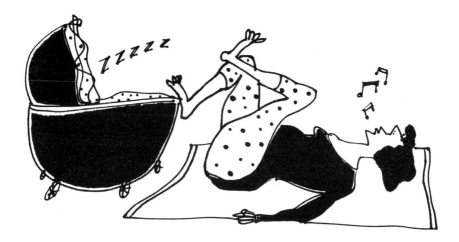

Exercise can help you bounce back after childbirth

Active living: plus points for men

1. Helps to reduce the risk of the single biggest cause of death in middle-aged men, heart disease. Regular vigorous activity can cut the risk by half.

2. Helps to overcome dependence on tobacco and alcohol.

3. Lets off steam and improves your ability to cope with stress.

4. Improves stamina, sex, and self-esteem. Helps keep you trim too.

Active living: plus points for children

1. Builds strong bones, joints and muscles.

2. Develops team spirit, leadership skills and the ability to get on with others.

3. Encourages active living as a lifelong habit.

4. Helps to discourage experimentation with cigarettes, solvents or drugs.

5. Gets the family doing things and enjoying life together.

Active living: plus points for older people

1. Improves the body's ability to resist illness.

2. Maintains muscle tone – important for mobility and independence.

3. Strengthens bones and joints – protects against injury from falls.

4. Improves quality of sleep.

5. Keeps you involved, meeting and interacting with other people.

6. Helps you feel good and able to show the young ones a thing or two.

Points to remember:

- Exercise and fun often go together.

- Age is no barrier and there are few medical conditions which can't be helped by being more active. If in doubt, consult your GP.

- Including exercise in your daily routine is easy and not time-consuming.

- The less fit you are, the sooner you'll feel the benefits.

- Build up your activities gradually – avoid the 'wham blam' mentality.

- Start being more active right now – make it a life-long, and long-life, habit.

WHAT IS FITNESS?

Fit for what?

In the simplest terms, being fit is being able to cope with the physical demands your life makes on you. Being strong enough to take the knocks and manage whatever lifting, shifting and carrying you may need to do without strain or injury. Being supple enough to reach those difficult places without pulling muscles or getting stiff, and having the stamina to keep going without collapsing in a breathless heap.

It's not the same thing as health, although it's an important aspect of it. And it's not a quest for absolute or total fitness. Even the most highly trained athlete never achieves that. There are always limits to fitness.

But whereas the athlete is trying to win, to be the champion – most of us are merely trying to survive, to cope with the slings and arrows of our everyday existence. Whilst the athlete hopes to achieve a sufficient level of fitness to give them the chance to 'go for gold', we need a sufficient level to enable us simply to get by as best as possible.

So fitness is relative – and the question for most of us is not so much 'Am I fit?', but 'Am I fit enough?'. Fit enough for everyday life, for the extra demands that happen from time to time, and for the longer-term protection against such threats as osteoporosis, high blood pressure and heart disease.

All of which leads to the more fundamental question, 'Am I active enough?' – not only to improve our fitness, important though that is, but also to gain the immediate benefits of feeling good, meeting people and having fun.

So, perhaps the word 'fitness' should be left to gym managers, PT instructors and exercise physiologists. Instead we should simply think in terms of our level of physical activity, and we should all try to move just that little bit more.

The S factors

Exercise takes many different forms, and affects the body in a variety of complex ways. But there are three main aspects of your physiology which regular activity can improve – stamina, suppleness and strength – collectively known as the 'S factors'.

Stamina

This is staying power – in other words, your ability to keep going, whether running, walking, swimming, cycling or other vigorous activity, without collapsing in a heap or gasping for breath. With enough stamina, your heart doesn't pound out of your chest, and your lungs don't feel as though they're bursting.

Stamina is useful when you have to dash up a flight or two of stairs, run for the bus or train, or keep up with the children. Stamina has beneficial effects on the heart and circulation. Regular exercise to maintain stamina can halve the risk of heart disease.

The best activities to improve stamina are fairly energetic (more than you're used to), make you slightly out of breath, and keep you moving for twenty minutes or more. This type of exercise is often called 'aerobic' exercise because, whilst you're doing it, you have to breathe in extra oxygen for your working muscles. Lots of the activities mentioned later in this chapter are good for stamina.

Suppleness

Suppleness is the ability to bend, stretch, twist and turn, using your joints to their full range, reaching all those awkward places. You need suppleness many times a day – for getting your clothes on and doing your hair, for getting in and out of the bath or the car, for travelling on buses or trains, for doing those fiddly jobs around the house. By keeping supple, you can not only manage these things, but you'll also be less likely to pull muscles and get stiff. Suppleness is particularly important as you get older. If muscles are not stretched regularly, they shorten, and in this way limit the movement of your joints.

Suppleness is achieved by activities or exercises that gently and gradually stretch your muscles and tighten your ligaments.

Strength

Being able to exert force – for pushing, pulling, lifting and shifting. You need strength all the time – to move around, carry shopping, climb upstairs, and take stubborn tops off bottles. It helps to protect you from sprains and strains. A strong back and tummy will help to maintain good posture.

Strength is built by using muscles against resistance – by doing the very things you need strength for – pushing, pulling, lifting and shifting. Many of the activities outlined below are good for building up your strength.

Activities and the S factors

Here's a rough and ready guide to the contribution various popular activities can make to the three S factors. Needless to say, what you get out of an activity depends very much on what you put in – a little extra effort can make a big difference. But in general, the more often you perform a physical task – any task – the more fully and completely your body and skills will adapt to cope with it. In fitness terms, this is known as the 'training effect'.

Activity	*Stamina*	*Suppleness*	*Strength*
Badminton	★★	★★★	★★
Climbing stairs	★★★	★	★★★
Cricket	★	★★	★★
Cycling (hard)	★★★★	★★	★★★
Dancing (ballroom)	★	★★★	★
Dancing (disco)	★★★	★★★★	★
Digging	★★★	★★	★★★★
Football	★★★	★★★	★★★
Golf	★★	★★	★
Hill walking	★★★	★	★★★
Housework	★	★★	★
Jogging	★★★★	★★	★★
Mowing the lawn	★★	★	★★★
Squash	★★★	★★★	★★★
Swimming (hard)	★★★★	★★★★	★★★★
Tennis	★★	★★★	★★
Walking (briskly)	★★★	★	★★
Weight-training	★	★	★★★★
Yoga	★	★★★★	★

Go for variety

As you can see from the chart, the different activities vary greatly in the ways they contribute to fitness, and there's much to be gained by mixing and matching so that you gain in all-round fitness. Compare the value of disco-dancing to hill-walking in terms of improving suppleness. Look at the difference between the value of digging compared to squash in improving strength. Even mowing the lawn or a good brisk walk compares favourably with some of the more obvious forms of exercise.

Exercise and your heart

Not only is regular aerobic activity a useful way to help you burn up calories, and hence lose weight, it also has a number of other beneficial effects that help to reduce the risk of heart disease.

It has a tonic effect on the balance of fatty substances in your blood, helping to remove cholesterol from your arteries and preventing atheromatous deposits that clog them.

It helps to reduce raised blood pressure. Although your blood pressure naturally rises during a bout of exercise or any physical exertion in order to force more blood into the working muscles, regular exercise has been shown to lower the resting blood pressure level. This is the blood pressure at rest, between exertions, which for most people is most of the time.

It's a useful way to combat stress. Research has found that regular, non-competitive, rhythmic aerobic activity – such as walking, running, swimming, dancing, skipping or cycling – helps to reduce the adrenalin and other stress hormones in the circulation, and stimulate endorphin (the pleasure hormone) in the brain.

And last but not least many smokers find that, by taking up a more active lifestyle, it's easier to cut down or give up the weed.

All in all, an active lifestyle with regular aerobic activity can reduce the risk of heart attack *by up to a half.*

Activity to beat osteoporosis

As we get beyond middle age, our bones become thinner, weaker and more fragile – a gradual process called osteoporosis. The obvious and all-too-common danger is the risk of fractures, particularly in old age. It happens to some extent to both sexes, but it's much more of a problem for women because it's worsened by their sudden loss of hormones during and after the menopause. Women also tend to have rather thinner and weaker bones to start with.

One of the best ways to beat osteoporosis is to take up an active lifestyle to help build up strong bones. Bones are not inert pieces of ivory, but living and constantly changing structures which have the ability to toughen up over a period of time in response to exercise. The best forms of activity are those that build up strength in the legs – walking is excellent for this. The earlier in life you become more active, the better, because the bones are better able to adapt when you're younger. But even in old age, they retain some powers of improvement – so, it's never too late.

Do I need a check-up?

Almost any activity is beneficial in some way – but it's important not to attempt things that are beyond your capacity. Most people, even older people, don't need a medical examination before becoming more active or taking up some form of exercise. If, however, you have hypertension (high blood pressure), a heart problem, chest trouble such as asthma or bronchitis, diabetes, arthritis or joint pains, severe back trouble, or you're recovering from an illness or operation, you should *consult your doctor*. In fact, appropriate activity is usually helpful for all these conditions, but it may have a bearing on your treatment, and it's best if your doctor knows about it and can discuss it with you.

Whatever activity you take up, always remember to start gently and build up gradually, day by day, week by week.

If you're over thirty-five you should have your blood pressure checked at least once every three years, *whether or not you're taking up a more active lifestyle.*

If you're pregnant there's no reason why you shouldn't keep up your favourite activities. Indeed, exercise is positively beneficial throughout pregnancy as long as it's comfortable. However, if you've suffered a miscarriage in a previous pregnancy, it's best to consult your doctor.

It's best not to exercise vigorously if you feel unwell. Wait until you feel better. You should also avoid vigorous exercise for at least an hour after a meal – to let the food get down, and prevent stomach cramp.

Stop what you're doing if you develop any of the following:

- pain
- dizziness
- feeling sick or unwell
- unusual fatigue.

If the problem doesn't settle after resting, see your doctor.

How fit are you?

Most people over-estimate their fitness and under-estimate their weight. This can cause a shock when they need to use their bodies in a different or more demanding way than they're used to. There's no single way of measuring your fitness, but answering these simple questions will give you some idea, albeit very approximate.

Do you quickly get short of breath walking uphill or even on the flat?

If yes, you really need to improve your stamina. Walking more is the best way to start.

Do your legs ache or feel weak after a few flights of stairs?

If yes, you need to build up your leg strength. A good way is to climb stairs more often!

Do you find it difficult to bend down to tie your shoelaces, or put your socks or tights on?

If yes, you need to improve your suppleness by daily stretching exercises and a more active way of life.

Is it difficult to reach awkward places on your body, combing the back of your hair for instance.

If yes, you need to develop more suppleness in your shoulders. Again, stretching exercsies are the answer.

Do you find it difficult to get out of a car, the bath or your armchair?

If yes, you need to improve the strength and suppleness in your arms and legs. You can do this by doing exercises or by taking up a suitable combination of the activities outlined later in this chapter.

A simple stamina test

If you can walk on the flat without difficulty, you could try the following simple test of stamina.

Time yourself walking or jogging (or a combination of both) for a distance of exactly one mile along a flat path or road, going as fast as you can *without letting yourself get uncomfortably short of breath*. It's likely to take between 10 and 20 minutes. Here's a rough guide to your stamina rating.

Minutes taken	Stamina rating
10 or under	very fit
10–12	quite fit
12–15	fair
15–20	rather unfit
20 or over	very unfit

These figures are based on averages for both sexes and all ages. Younger people (under thirty-five) should be able to do better, and should therefore grade themselves in the next category down. Older people (over fifty-five) should grade themselves in the next category up.

Many health centres, clubs and gyms offer more elaborate and accurate fitness tests, covering stamina, suppleness and strength. Ideally, they should be combined with individual advice on the best forms of exercise for you.

But, the fact is that you don't need any kind of fitness test in order to take up a more active lifestyle – nor to feel the benefits.

HOW MUCH? HOW OFTEN?

There's no pat answer to either of these questions. It all depends. It depends on how active you are at present, and how fit. It depends on what you're hoping to achieve, whether it be a particular level of fitness or a more active way of life.

Broadly speaking, any activity is better than none – and if you do a little more than you're used to, that's even better. The important principle is to make exercise part and parcel of your everyday existence, rather than a 'programme' that you have to force yourself into.

So it's partly a matter of finding activities you enjoy, and getting into them with vim and vigour, and partly finding more physical ways of doing the things you usually do.

To gain real benefit for your heart it's important to choose activities which are sufficiently energetic to make you mildly short of breath and to continue them for either about ten minutes a day, or at least twenty minutes three times a week. Walking, running, dancing, skipping, swimming, cycling, jogging on-the-spot – any of these aerobic activities will do the trick.

Take your time

It takes time to adapt to a more active way of life, so don't rush at it. Always start gently and build up gradually, day by day, week by week.

Warming-up and cooling-down

If you're going to do something quite vigorous, it's sensible to do a few simple stretching exercises first to 'warm up' your muscles – particularly calf stretches and hamstring stretches. This helps to avoid sprains and strains. Similarly, after vigorous exercise you should take a few minutes to cool down slowly by jogging gently and then walking about a little. This helps to avoid stiffness.

If it hurts, you're doing it wrong

Don't believe the person who tells you 'there's no gain without pain'. This is a dangerous myth. To be of benefit to health and well-being, physical activity should be enjoyable, not uncomfortable. And certainly not painful. Never push yourself so hard that exercise becomes unpleasant.

Keep it up

Many of the benefits of active living are long term – a healthier heart, stronger bones and a leaner, lither figure. This means that you need to keep active for years, for decades, for life. Unfortunately, if you stop exercising, the benefits will soon melt away. The slide from peak fitness to a gasping heap takes a mere six weeks or so. You can't put fitness in the bank.

But for each week that you stay active, not only will it be another week of feeling good, but also another week in which the insidious processes leading to heart disease or osteoporosis are stopped in their tracks.

Golden Opportunities

You don't need to be a fanatic to keep the body in order. Start by looking out for more physical ways of doing things.

- Take the stairs instead of the lift. Start by walking downstairs first. If it's too far to go upstairs, climb a few floors then use the lift. Gradually increase the number of floors.
- Walk to the shops and only use the bus to come back. Stride out and get there faster. Spend the bus fare you've saved on a trip to the leisure centre.
- Walk to the post box – and walk back again.
- Keep up with the kids. Run them about a bit.
- Let the dog take you for a walk more often.

Points to remember:

- Exercise can be great fun and need not be formalised.
- Getting started is not as difficult as you might think – just do it.
- Build it up slowly and gradually – avoid the 'wham blam' approach.
- Know your limits, particularly if you have a medical condition.
- Prepare yourself, use the correct equipment and clothes.
- Try to fit it in with your lifestyle.
- Experiment. Try something new that appeals to you.
- Share the experience with others.
- There's no short cut – you've just got to keep moving.
- You can't put fitness in the bank.

HOW TO GET STARTED

If you're not very active at the moment, perhaps rather unfit, or, less than enthusiastic about physical exertion, you may feel somewhat daunted at the prospect of throwing yourself into a new life of leaps, bounds and physical jerks.

But that's not the way to go about it. Becoming more active doesn't have to mean a single leap or bound if you don't want it to, and you may never meet a physical jerk. Getting started doesn't have to be at all difficult. You simply do what you like, as long as it's a little more physically demanding than you're used to. Later, as you get fitter, you might be tempted to try the more fancy stuff.

But throwing yourself at it, wham-blam, hammer-and-tongs is nearly always a mistake. This evangelical approach to exercise may be dramatic but is usually short-lived, and tends to produce a string of horror stories – pulled muscles, strained ligaments, wrecked backs, and perhaps worse. By contrast, easing yourself into a more active existence should be a subtle process, a change of attitude that grows within you, not something you force on yourself. It's a life-long affair and has little to do with the sporty stereotype, tracksuit or otherwise. So, always start gently and build up slowly.

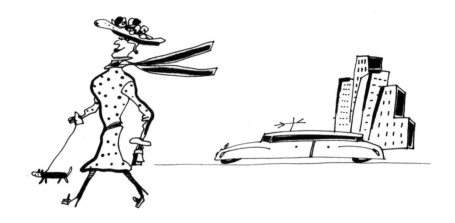

Give the car a rest – get walking

Be prepared

Making a bit more physical effort in your daily life doesn't require much preparation – perhaps a raincoat or brolly if you're walking to the shops or station, or keeping your swimming things in your cupboard at work so that you can have a lunch-time dip. But, for more organised activities, it pays to have the basic gear.

Clothing

The good news is that most activities don't require any expensive clothes or footwear. Generally, sensible light comfortable clothes and strong shoes such as trainers are all that are needed.

If you intend to do a fair bit of activity out of doors on a hot, sunny day, it's a good idea to invest in a light hat that will shade you from the sun and keep off the rain. A white hat bobbing up and down is also hard to miss by vehicle drivers.

Your clothing should be light and loose enough to allow you to remain cool, and made of a natural fibre such as cotton rather than synthetic. In cold weather, many thin loose layers are better than a few thick ones – you can peel them off, one by one, as you warm up. A brightly-coloured top will help you to be seen on the roads, particularly at night.

For women, a good supportive bra is important, but it shouldn't be so tight that it restricts breathing.

In warm weather or indoors, shorts are more comfortable than trousers – but it's useful to be able to slip on a pair of tracksuit bottoms after vigorous exercise to prevent too rapid cooling and stiffness. Men need supportive underpants or, for more vigorous activities, a jockstrap.

Footwear

If we believed all those sleek, scientific commercials, we might be forgiven for thinking that there's no point in taking another step without being shod with a pair of dyna-spring, mega-thrust, ultra-cushioned, pro-zoom trainers – or what we used to call plimsolls.

While expensive, specialised footwear may be essential for the dedicated athlete, we mere mortals can get by quite nicely with far less expense. Nevertheless, it's worth choosing with some care. Look for a good thick heel to protect the sole from the shock of repeatedly hitting hard ground. A strong arch support is also desirable.

You'll notice that your shoes always feel tighter at the end of exercising than they did beforehand. This is because your feet spread and swell slightly. A size larger than your normal footwear can help and will allow for wearing woollen socks in cold weather.

Choosing activities

Such is the interest in exercise and activity that the past few years have seen an explosion in the number of leisure centres, health clubs, sports facilities and gyms. The choice today is enormous, and this is all to the good. And yet, for many enjoyable activities, all that's needed is some open space, indoors or out, and the will to make use of it.

Try to choose activities which:

- fit in with your lifestyle

- you enjoy

- you can do frequently

- are conveniently close to home or to work

- are fairly weatherproof

- are appropriate to your physical condition

Walking

Walking is an ideal way to introduce yourself to activity particularly if you have neglected exercise for some time. Gradually build up the distance and the speed so that it makes you slightly breathless. Look for opportunities to walk instead of using the bus, car or lift.

If you intend to walk for an extended period, carry out some warm-up exercises first. Gentle bends and stretches help avoid muscle and tendon damage. If you'll be walking in the hills, remember to tell someone where you are going, and take suitable protective clothing for a sudden change in the weather. It's a good idea to seek expert advice about the area in which you intend to walk.

Activity value

Walking is not only excellent for relieving stress and tension but also increases stamina and strength in the legs. It's less good for improving suppleness, but there's no reason why you shouldn't pause on the walk for a few minutes of bending and stretching.

Jogging and running

A step up in commitment, jogging or running is an excellent aerobic activity for those who are already reasonably fit. There's some risk of jarring injuries to the heels, ankles and knees, much reduced by wearing good running shoes and keeping to soft surfaces like grass. For those who run on roads, there's the constant danger of traffic – so make sure you put on something bright and reflective, especially in poor light. Work up gradually to greater distances and speeds, with plenty of walking rests.

Activity value

Excellent for stamina but little else. Avoid this form of exercise if you have arthritis in your back, hips, knees or feet, or are very overweight. Consider cycling or swimming instead.

Swimming

Often considered the best form of activity for all round fitness, swimming is cheap and enjoyable for all the family. Many pools have special sessions for the over-fifties, adults only, or other particular groups, and it doesn't cost a great deal. There are often special rates for people on lower incomes. An ability to swim with confidence can lead on to more adventurous sports such as scuba diving, wind surfing or water-skiing. These are not so cheap.

Activity value

If you work hard enough at it, and don't just pootle about, swimming can be excellent for all three S-factors: stamina, strength and suppleness. It's marvellous if you're overweight, have arthritis or back problems or some disability, because the water supports you. The only snags are that you have to undress, and get wet.

Cycling

The bike is a wonderfully low-tech, ecologically sound, wind-in-your-hair way of going places, fast. It's a particularly rapid means of transit in the city, often beating cars and buses over the shorter distances. It's easy to park, and it'll carry a fair amount of clobber. The main disadvantages are that you can get rather wet in the rain, you have to watch out for potholes, and have eyes in the back of your head for drivers who have scant regard for cyclists.

Bike styles and prices vary greatly, but for town work choose a machine with straight handlebars which allow good vision and control. Always wear a sturdy helmet and bright reflective clothes or sashes. Waterproof gear is essential if there's a chance of rain. Buy the biggest and the best lights you can afford – it's money very well spent.

Amazingly, children don't consider cycling as exercise and will usually agree to a family outing. Choose somewhere safe so you can relax while you ride. It's a good idea to encourage your children to take a cycling proficiency test.

Activity value

Stamina is the great bonus from cycling, providing you push hard enough to get yourself mildly breathless. Leg strength is improved but there is no marked effect upon suppleness. If you can use a bike for all, or even part, of your journey to work, it's a superb way of fitting exercise into your daily routine.

Bowling

Traditional bowls is mainly an outdoor pursuit, although indoor greens have been established. Ten pin bowling is now very popular and most towns have a bowling alley. Continental travel has brought the closely related sport of boules, an outdoor game that can be played on any flat ground or sand. All of these games provide relatively gentle exercise and an opportunity to meet and chat. Age is no barrier, many towns and villages have greens and club fees are generally inexpensive.

Activity value

Bowling is a good excuse for reaching and stretching to improve shoulder suppleness. The bending and crouching helps to build strength in the legs, without jarring the joints. Unfortunately bowling does nothing for stamina.

Golf

An increasingly popular sport, although it can still be expensive and difficult to join a private club. Fortunately, many local authorities have public courses which are quite cheap and often very good. You can hire a set of clubs to try your hand. If you get to like the game, you can usually pick up a second-hand half-set quite cheaply. You'll also need comfortable, waterproof shoes and an umbrella.

Activity value

Like many other activities the amount you get out is related to the effort you put in. As long as you pull your trolley or carry your clubs, it can be surprisingly energetic – a full round being four or five miles, perhaps up and down slopes. Good for stamina and leg strength.

Badminton

Great fun, even for beginners. Lots of reaching and jumping, power shots and deftly subtle ones. Like all racquet games, it exercises your brain as well as your body. Badminton can be played indoors or out, needing very little space – facilities are everywhere. A good racquet needn't be expensive. You'll also need good supportive shoes.

Activity value

Good all round exercise for suppleness of shoulder and back, strength of legs, and stamina. All the more enjoyable if you play doubles.

Tennis

Fast moving and fun, tennis can be sociable, challenging and the ideal family game. Hiring a municipal court is not expensive. Joining a private club usually is. A good racquet doesn't come cheap either, but you can probably borrow or hire one to start with.

Activity value

Like badminton, tennis can really stretch you and make you run your socks off. As with badminton, good supportive shoes are a must.

Squash

Squash has a reputation for being highly competitive and physically very demanding. You have to be fit to play squash – so don't think of it as a way of getting fit. It's all sudden bursts of energy, deep reaches, power shots and not a little aggression. There's some risk of being hit by the fast-moving ball or racquet. Think twice about taking it up in middle age. Start very gently however old you are. It's played mostly in private clubs, which are pricey – but more and more leisure centres have courts for hire.

Activity value

Once you have attained a fair level of fitness, squash is a fun way of maintaining it. It's excellent for all three S-factors.

Dance

You may not think of dance as exercise – but it certainly is. Most forms of dance – rock, modern, tap, or folk, for example – can be very energetic. Even ballroom and 'old time' dancing can involve a lot of stretching, turning and striding around the dance-floor. Moving to music is one of life's real pleasures, and a great chance to socialise. If you don't know the steps, your local leisure centre, dance studio or adult education institute may run inexpensive classes.

Activity value

Depending on how much you put into it, dancing can be particularly good for improving suppleness and stamina. It's a great excuse for doing aerobic exercise to music, without realising that you're keeping fit. What's more, it's good for your soul as well as your body.

Keep fit, aerobics, and work-out classes

If you like being with others, exercise classes offer a great opportunity to commit yourself to regular activity. They're fun and fulfilling, helping to motivate you into the exercise habit. They're also a good way of meeting people.

It's important to start at the right level for you -and not attempt anything you don't think you could do without discomfort. Almost every community has an exercise class of some sort. Those run by your local leisure centre or adult education institute will not be expensive.

Activity value

Excellent for all-round fitness – stamina, suppleness, and strength – and for slimming. Good for contouring tummy, hips and thighs.

Weight-training

Don't worry, you won't end up like a Sumo wrestler! Training with weights is not the same as weight-lifting. The essence of weight-training is repetitive movements using light handweights or gym machines with levers and pulleys.

So, it's simply an extension of on-the-spot strength exercises. It's also suitable for many people with a disability.

Even so, because of the greater forces involved, you need to know how to work with weights properly. Your local leisure or sports centre, or fitness club, is just the place for advice and supervision. Most of the equipment would not look out of place in the Tower of London, but many people find it relaxing and even hypnotic. Try it out first before you think of buying any expensive equipment. The small ads are full of unwanted items bought in a moment of misguided enthusiasm.

Activity value
Like swimming, weight training, used in the correct manner, can improve all the S factors – stamina, suppleness and strength – particularly strength. Excellent for contouring tummy, hips and thighs. However, you can hurt yourself if you don't learn how to lift correctly.

Judo and martial arts
Judo, karate, kung fu, jiujitsu, aikido, kendo and other martial arts are physically quite demanding activities, particularly suitable for younger people. They have increased enormously in popularity, especially among women who wish to be able to defend themselves against attack. As with all contact sports, there's some risk of injury – but with proper facilities, training and supervision, this should be minimal.

Activity value
Good for strength and suppleness. Less good for stamina.

Yoga
In yoga you learn to relax by deep breathing and gentle control of your movements. There are various forms of yoga – some more holistic than others. All involve moving to certain poses or positions which stretch particular muscle groups. You can also learn to meditate.

Yoga is suitable for all ages, and there are lots of classes available at low cost.

Activity value

Excellent for suppleness and relaxation. Also good for strengthening the back and tummy muscles. But it does nothing for stamina.

Sports and leisure centres

These centres, with their wide range of facilities and classes, have really blossomed over the past few years. Forget the idea that these places are temples for the super-fit and ultra-athletic. They may have been once, but not any more. These days there's something for everybody – people of all ages, shapes, sizes and physical ability. One thing is certain, you will not feel out of place or out of pocket when you go along to your local sports or leisure centre.

In some areas they have taken on the role of community centres and provide a great deal more than just sports and recreation. Reduced prices are usually available for retired or unemployed people, and those on a low income.

ACTION POINTS

- getting started is not as hard as you think – just do a little more than you're used to – something you enjoy. The choice is enormous.

- if you like company, get family or friends to join in.

- you don't need expensive equipment to be more active –just sensible clothing and footwear.

- most people don't need to see their doctor first. But if you have a medical condition that may be affected by energetic exercise, seek your GP's advice.

- check out your local leisure centre and park – there are lots of opportunities there for everybody, whatever shape you're in.

- have fun and keep moving!

FEELING GOOD

SHEER PLEASURE

There's an old saying that when an optimist and a pessimist see half a glass of beer, the pessimist says it's half empty, but the optimist says it's half full. As a result of this way of thinking, the optimist is not only likely to enjoy life more, but may also have a longer life to enjoy.

There's increasing evidence that people who look on the bright side of life do seem to be able to shrug off illnesses more easily and have a better chance of beating chronic diseases. Recently, medical science has confirmed that a positive attitude promotes health. Tests have shown that positive thoughts stimulate the release of certain brain hormones, endorphins and enkephalins, which are the body's own in-built version of morphine. The resulting feelings of pleasure, satisfaction and happiness are combined with a higher threshold to pain. In other words you feel good and are less susceptible to discomfort and distress.

What's more, these feelings not only help people to cope with disease, but, in some cases, may even delay the disease process itself.

Take cancer, for example. Studies have shown that people who have a positive optimistic fighting attitude to their cancer are more likely to achieve a cure, or survive longer. There's even some evidence that positive thinking can help to prevent some cancers from appearing in the first place.

This is all very well, but how can you feel positive and happy if you're under stress, or depressed, or in pain, or otherwise miserable? You can't just wave a magic wand and suddenly see everything through rose-tinted specs.

True. But you would be surprised how much positive thinking you can muster if you make a bit of an effort – especially if family and friends rally round too.

Sharing your worries, sorting out problems into aspects that aren't too daunting, finding the positive side of things, putting on a brave face, taking a bit more control of your life, finding time to relax, doing things you enjoy, having a good old laugh, helping others, embracing religion – all of these can really make a big difference.

So many of life's ills – social, mental and physical – stem from negative feelings – resentment, hatred, lack of confidence, low self-esteem. If we can learn to understand what makes us feel good as well as bad, and can find ways of enhancing our lives without becoming too much of a burden to others, we'll all be a lot healthier.

STRESS

We all use the word 'stress' a great deal. We live in a 'stressful' society. Life is full of 'stresses'. There are times when each and every one of us feels 'stressed out'.

And yet, in strictly medical terms, there's no such thing as 'stress'. It's a lay-person's expression to describe the whole welter of pressures, worries, concerns, anxieties, fears, and the mental and physical toll they take of us.

The effects of stress can certainly be real enough: the frantic mother of three young children who gets tension headaches; or the factory worker made redundant after seventeen years' loyal service who gets a duodenal ulcer; or the teenager who takes an overdose because her only true love has dumped her; or the husband sinking deeper into an affair and drinking larger and larger scotches; or the older woman battling with the menopause who slumps into depression. All of these, and countless others, are manifestations of stress.

Is stress normal?

Yes and no. It's perfectly normal for us all to feel stressed from time to time. It's part of everyday life. For many people the urgency of deadlines or the pressure of work can be invigorating and exciting. But one person's stimulation is another's strain. If the pressure becomes a burden that get's on top of you, and you feel trapped, inadequate or ground down, then the stress can lead to all sorts of health problems.

Signs of stress

Most problems are those caused by a person's response to the anxiety. They may, for instance, smoke too many cigarettes, or drink too much, or eat too much, or get into arguments, or become violent, or make mistakes, or take drugs.

As stress builds up, there are recognisable changes in behaviour, such as:

- Constant fatigue and poor sleep patterns.
- Poor concentration and short-term memory. Difficulty in following long conversations.
- Increasing introspection. Only matters of direct relevance to the stress factors: earning money, meeting deadlines, getting to appointments, etc. appear important.
- Personal and family neglect. Personal appearance becomes irrelevant. Children and partners become obstructions rather than assets for pleasure.
- Repetitive behaviour. Checking and rechecking things several times – Is the alarm set? Are the dishes clean? Have the kids done their homework? Did I bring the right files?
- Eating too much or too little.
- Increasing irritability. A 'short fuse' needing very little to spark off an aggressive reaction.
- Abuse of alcohol or even drugs.

Bodily changes

The other main group of problems related to stress are psychosomatic – physical illnesses brought on by psychological stress, such as headaches, insomnia, skin rashes, asthma, high blood pressure, nausea, irritable bowels, aches and pains,

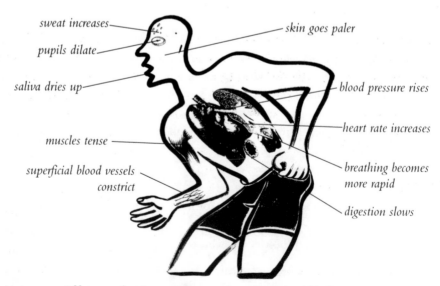

Effects of acute stress – the 'fight or flight' reaction

and many other common problems. In the longer term it can trigger more serious illnesses such as peptic ulcers, colitis, strokes and heart attacks.

Coping with stress

Most of us recognise stress when we're suffering it. We usually know when things are getting on top of us, or when we're getting far too tense. And if we don't recognise it in ourselves, other people usually spot the signs and symptoms pretty early on – an inability to relax, constant anxiety, grinding teeth, white knuckles, short temper, and any of the other horrors we've already considered.

Obviously your personality has a lot to do with stressful situations. You may be really cool under pressure – or a bundle of nerves. You may have a devil-may-care attitude – or desperately try to do the 'right thing'. You may thrive on huge responsibilities and constant deadlines – or go into a blind panic. But oddly enough, it's often the very people who like to be in control, who like to take responsibility and get things properly organised, who are most vulnerable to stress, anxiety and breakdown when things go badly wrong in a way that they can't handle.

Crisis – what crisis?

The first step is to recognise stress in your life. It means asking yourself a few very fundamental questions such as:

- What are the most important things in my life? My family? My friends? My job? My hobbies? My health?
- How much time should I give to my real priorities?
- How much time do I have to myself?
- How can I manage my time better?
- How can I parcel out my tasks more efficiently?
- Do I really need to do everything I think I need to do?
- Can I find someone else to help shoulder my burdens?
- Can I sort out just one problem for now?

You may find that by standing back for a moment and reappraising your life and the way you run it (or it runs you) you can make a few adjustments that pay huge dividends in reducing stress. Of course, many of us have such major worries that there may seem to be no easy answers. But usually, by thinking about as many options as you can, and by talking them over with someone you feel at ease with, you'll find that solutions begin to present themselves, that a way through the quagmire begins to emerge.

The fight or flight reaction

When you're frightened, excited or stimulated to take some nerve-racking action, your adrenal glands, just above your kidneys, produce a hormone called adrenalin. To exert its effect, adrenalin has to travel throughout the body in the bloodstream. Its first stop is the heart, where it increases the pulse rate and blood pressure in order to get more blood to the brain and muscles.

Adrenalin also has many other effects. For instance, it inhibits the salivary glands, causing the characteristic dry mouth. It diverts blood from the skin, making it go pale. It stimulates the release of glucose into the bloodstream to supply the muscles with instant energy. And it dilates the pupils of the eyes to let in more light.

In simple biological terms, when your body reacts in this way it's ready to take action either by fighting or running away. You are experiencing the "fight or flight" reaction, and, even in this day and age it could save your life if you ever had to leap out of the way of a maniacal messenger-bike.

Stress triggers

One way to minimise the damage stress is causing you is to learn to recognise 'stress triggers' – everyday situations that really wind you up and bring on stressful feelings or bodily reactions – and to find ways of defusing them.

Examples are endless – long check-out queues, late buses, traffic snarl-ups, panics about getting things done, screaming kids, irritating in-laws, noisy neighbours, unreliable workmates, and so on *ad infinitem*. Situations like these will never go away, but recognising them as stress triggers and coping with them is halfway to reducing their effects.

How you cope with them may not be so easy of course. It requires a considerable effort of will to control your irritation or anxiety. You have to tell yourself to stay calm and find some distraction or diversion, some way round the problem.

For instance, when the traffic is making you tense, try looking out of the window and simply give somebody a smile to show camaraderie for a common problem. Now is your chance to have a good stretch and shift your bottom in the seat. When minor things occur which would normally annoy and stress you – the engaged phone, the bus that sails on past your out-stretched arm, the screw that drops between the floorboards – adopt a Zen attitude and recognise that these are all trivia. Watch how other people react, some will stamp and curse over so little, while others will give a sideways grin. Who will live longer?

You can also help yourself by using some of the simple relaxation techniques described below.

ANXIETY AND TENSION

Anxiety, like fire, can be a good servant but a bad master. We need anxiety to help us out of sticky situations. Without anxiety our ancestors would have been quickly gobbled up by sabre-toothed tigers. But too much anxiety is itself a killer. It eats away at our mind and body. It drives us to smoke, drink and other potentially destructive acts. It interferes with work and wrecks relationships. Anxiety, like fire, has to be confronted and controlled.

What is anxiety?

It's a form of fear – sometimes with an obvious clear-cut cause such as money worries, family stresses, work problems, concern about physical health, phobias – but often for no apparent reason. Even so, by its very nature, anxiety often fuels even more fear. A vicious cycle may be established where fear breeds fear in a spiral of anxiety. Such spirals can result in panic attacks or, in more chronic form, physical illnesses such as eczema, asthma, peptic ulcers and even heart attacks.

Bodily tension

One response to this fear is tension. Muscles contract, blood pressure rises, the heart beats faster and perhaps irregularly, causing palpitations. In themselves harmless, these symptoms can be frightening, increasing the anxiety and tension still further. The person breathes rapidly, which combined with the muscle tension, can make their chest feel tight, even painful. It can also cause a tingling sensation, particularly down the arms and legs. All this convinces many sufferers, and quite a few doctors, that they're having a heart attack. But, in fact, it's hyperventilation syndrome, often linked to a panic attack.

PANIC ATTACKS

A vortex of horror, a dreadful mounting fear that feeds on itself, an unbearable, unstoppable, sheer blind terror. Words can't describe the awful nature of a panic attack. They are suffered by at least one person in thirty at some time in their lives, many more women than men; once experienced, never forgotten.

What's the cause?

All of us have had moments of intense fear or even panic. Childhood is filled with frights – imagined or real. Later, many of us develop phobias – usually to such things as snakes, mice, heights, or confined spaces. But panic attacks seem to be something different. Instead of having the horrors about a particular object or situation, panic attack sufferers get panicky about panic itself. It's a dreadful fear of fear – afraid of being afraid.

As their terror mounts, their heart pounds in their chest, their skin blanches and breaks into a cold sweat, their breathing becomes rapid and shallow, and their head spins. But, merciful release though it would be, they usually don't pass out.

But there must be some reason for it

The reason varies from person to person. Some doctors believe it's linked to premenstrual syndrome, others to the menopause, still others to general stress or anxiety. It may also be the product of an obsessive or compulsive personality. There's a well-recognised link between panic attacks and agoraphobia – the fear of going out, especially to public places – but which comes first, the panic attacks or the agoraphobia, is often none too clear. Certainly for someone who's had a panic attack, agoraphobia may be just around the corner.

What triggers an attack?

Usually it's being in the same sort of situation they were when they had their first panic. For most sufferers it's finding themselves in some crowded place – a shop, a bus queue, a gathering – with a feeling of being trapped, exposed, or horribly embarrassed – and this is enough to trigger the terror.

How long do they last?

Each attack only lasts minutes, although it seems like a lifetime. They tend to come in spates, every few days for maybe two or three weeks. But they may be much fewer and further between, and keep occurring for months or years. There's no fixed pattern.

They do tend to be linked to the sufferer's general level of anxiety or stress. Often they fade away as circumstances improve – a happier relationship, a change of job, better living accommodation, children starting school.

How can panic attacks be beaten?

The first and most difficult thing is to recognise that the fear is coming from within, and not from the trigger situation itself. Although the sufferer may accept this as the rational truth, they are likely to find it hard to accept emotionally.

Family and friends can help by understanding the problem, and by helping the person to feel calm and unflustered, and not made to feel a nuisance. Just being there with the sufferer in a potential trigger situation can provide security and reassurance.

What's the treatment?

The only way positively to beat panic attacks is to learn how to confront the fear and see it off. This means the sufferer has to build up enough trust in his or her ability to handle the anxiety, working in easy stages to gain confidence and control the fear.

One of the most effective forms of help is a combination of relaxation techniques and behavioural therapy. Deep breathing and auto-suggestion can maintain calmness whilst the sufferer, together with the psychotherapist, deliberately faces increasingly difficult situations over a period of several weeks, until the bogey of panic is finally exorcised.

Unfortunately, there aren't enough psychotherapists available on the NHS, and most sufferers seeking treatment have to find one privately.

Self-help

1. Learn to understand your panic, and that it's fear of fear itself.

2. Find ways of building up your self-confidence – any way will help.

3. Learn simple techniques to help yourself relax. There are lots of paperback books to tell you how.

5. Don't run away from difficult situations – force yourself to brave them if only for a few minutes to begin with.

6. Find a psychotherapist to help you build up your ability to withstand fear.

PHOBIAS

If the thought of spiders makes you shudder, you're not alone. Arachnophobia is one of the most common phobias – along with fear of cats, worms, bats and mice.

But even more frequent are the more general phobias, such as fear of enclosed spaces (claustrophobia), fear of heights and, the commonest and most crippling of all, agoraphobia – fear of going out and about.

Fear becomes a phobia when it's excessive and irrational, often leading to acute anxiety and panic. About one person in ten has some sort of deep-seated fear or loathing that amounts to a phobia. But only a small proportion has it badly enough to seek help.

Women seem to have a greater tendency towards phobias than men – perhaps linked to in-built differences in their emotional make-up. Most phobias stem from childhood scares – perhaps being shut in a dark cupboard, being startled by the sudden movement of a mouse, or terrified by a thunderstorm. Sometimes a phobia is 'learned' from another member of the family.

Agoraphobia is rather different. It usually starts in a person's twenties or early thirties and is twice as common in women. It's almost invariably linked to panic attacks, often brought on by premenstrual tension.

Phobias can be conquered only by facing the fear head on, instead of always running away from it. The most effective treatment is called desensitisation and involves getting used to the feared object or situation in gradual step-by-step stages.

If you're an arachnophobe, for instance, you'd first spend time simply talking to someone (preferably a trained psychotherapist) about spiders. Then you'd look at pictures of the little horrors and describe them in detail. Next, you'd get used to looking at a dead spider in a jam-jar with the lid on. Then with the lid off. Then with the dead spider in your hand. Then, a live spider in the jar with the lid on, and off. Finally, you end up holding the live spider in your hand – and at the same time you smile.

This whole process may take three sessions or twenty, but it's helped thousands of people to overcome their crippling phobia.

On a short fuse

A hunted or hurt animal will act unpredictably and out of character. Not surprisingly, a person under stress, feeling insecure or worried, may react to people with an uncharacteristic irritation or even anger. Recognising this reaction in someone close is part of being a good friend, and requires tolerance and understanding.

For the anxious person, even the simplest of things can lead to irritation and avoidance. Letters and bills, for example, become insurmountable obstacles. Attempts by family or friends to draw attention to the problem are often met with unjustified wrath. From these small beginnings can come the major rows which often end up in disastrous splits and schisms.

Nervous breakdown

Sudden floods of tears, screaming fits, inability to make any decisions, exhaustion, insomnia, bursts of uncontrollable anger – there are all sorts of ways people may react when they've reached the end of their tether. They get to a point when it's just all too much for them, and something snaps. Quite suddenly, they can no longer function normally. They're having a 'nervous breakdown'.

In fact the term has no real medical or psychiatric meaning – but it's a familiar way of describing various sorts of mental crisis that are usually triggered by stress. Often the stress is linked to severe anxiety, loss or bereavement. Overwhelming family problems, pressures of work, redundancy, loss of a loved one – these are some of the ordeals that can cause a vulnerable person to crack up and find themselves unable to cope or carry on.

Although no one is immune to a nervous breakdown if the stress is great enough, the most vulnerable people tend to be the worriers, who churn things over, the perfectionists who like to get things right, and the obsessives who are creatures of habit. Obviously, there are some of these traits in all of us, but many people are ruled by a mind-set that can all too easily be knocked off its tracks by adverse circumstances.

Even more vulnerable are those who are already emotionally strained or who have a pre-existing mental illness. If, for instance, someone is subject to mood swings, with manic highs and dismal lows, or has suffered the horror of panic attacks or phobias, or has had symptoms of chronic anxiety for some time, they are living on a knife-edge and much more likely to be pushed to the limit by some stressful event or situation.

The greatest danger is that, in a fit of desperation or self-reproach, the person having a breakdown might try to do him or herself some harm, perhaps even attempt suicide. Fortunately, this extreme reaction is fairly unusual – but watch out for the warning signs. If people talk of being a burden, of being trapped, of wanting to escape, or of hating themselves – it might be the only clue you get before they do something awful. Needless to say, lesser disasters are much more likely – wrecked relationships, family break-ups, ruined careers, financial crises. Many people come through a nervous breakdown only to find that their lives are never quite the same again.

The first thing is to recognise that all is not well and that the person you know and love can no longer cope. In its early stages, a breakdown may not always be obvious – but if they are suddenly tearful at inappropriate moments, become agitated or fearful for no obvious reason, are paralysed by indecision, can't concentrate on anything, lose all motivation, feel drained of energy, suffer inexplicable panics, or suddenly start behaving abnormally in some other way, then the signs are there. It's important that family, friends and workmates do their best to be sympathetic, understanding and supportive at this time of crisis.

People suffering a breakdown often don't recognise it themselves and may have to be persuaded to seek help. More often than not it's another member of the family or a friend who first alerts the GP to the problem. If necessary, the sufferer may be referred to a counsellor or psychiatrist.

Telephone helplines may play a vital part in averting a breakdown by helping people cope with severe stress, and pointing them in the direction of professional advice and treatment.

The greatest benefit may come from taking time off work, having a holiday, or learning to relax and conquer the symptoms of stress. But many people who have had a breakdown need psychiatric treatment in the form of psychotherapy or medication. Some may need to be admitted to a psychiatric unit for full assessment and treatment.

JUST YOU RELAX

Even if your life is reasonably under control, there are bound to be moments which really wind you up and make you very tense indeed. It might be contemplating an important meeting, an emotional occasion, a performance, facing a family crisis, sitting in a traffic jam, or any of so many stressful situations. It might be the culmination of a particularly tough day or week, or the few awful days before your period.

Whatever the cause of the tension, there are ways in which you can use your mind and body to help ease it away. In short, you can learn to relax.

Relaxation techniques

There are many different approaches, but they all use either the body to calm the mind, or the mind to relax the body.

Deep breathing

When you're really tense, you take rapid, shallow breaths through your mouth, using the upper part of your chest. But by breathing slowly and deeply through your nose, using your diaphragm, you can ease away tension.

Lie or sit comfortably, preferably in a quiet place, with your eyes shut. Start by taking in a very long, steady breath, right into every corner of your lungs. Hold it for a few seconds and then let it out very slowly without forcing any of it. Just relax, and let the air flow out under its own momentum.

With the next breath, don't deliberately breathe in, let it happen naturally, only as deeply as it wants to. Hold it – and relax. And the same again. And again. After a few breaths, you'll notice that your chest is doing less and less of the work and your tummy more and more. Eventually, with each breath, your tummy bulges slightly, and your chest doesn't move at all. This is deep abdominal breathing. Very relaxing.

Serene thoughts

In the same way that it's possible to become tense and nervous just by *imagining* some awful threat, it's quite possible to calm yourself by imagining something soothing and tranquil.

Make yourself as comfortable as possible, shut your eyes, and try to imagine a scene that conjures up a feeling of serenity for you: perhaps waves lapping on a sun-drenched beach, or a waterfall, or a place in the country with the sound of rustling leaves and birdsong. Imagine the whole scene in detail and imagine yourself there. Wallow in the scene for as long as you can spare. This is best combined with deep breathing.

Progressive relaxation

This technique relies first on tensing, and then on relaxing, groups of muscles, progressing from toes to head. It can be added to deep breathing and serene thoughts.

Again, lie or sit comfortably in a quiet place, and shut your eyes. Place your legs slightly apart and your arms a little away from your sides. Now, without moving your legs, pull your toes up towards your face, tensing the muscles at the front of your calves. Feel the tension for a few seconds, and then relax. Let the tension drain away. Now, do the same thing with the muscles at the front of your thighs by forcing your knees back and tightening your kneecaps. Feel the tension, and then relax. Let it drain away. Then do it with your tummy muscles. Then your forearm muscles, by clenching your fists. Then your neck by hunching your shoulders. And finally screw your face into a tight wince, as if someone was about to pop a balloon right in front of your nose. And then relax. Just breathe deeply for a few minutes and let all the tension drain away.

Meditation

Don't be put off by any preconceived ideas about flower-power or psychodelia. Meditation has been practised for centuries, especially in the Orient, and is a remarkably effective way of achieving inner calm. It takes deep breathing, serene thoughts and progressive relaxation a stage further.

Lie or sit comfortably in a quiet place. Close your eyes. After a minute or so of deep breathing, and relaxing from the feet upwards, focus your mind's eye on a point between your two eyes, keeping them shut. Think of this point as a tunnel. Now let the tunnel draw you into it. Let it suck you in at an accelerating pace. Let it pull all your bodily tension through it into the far distance. Some people also hum an 'mmmmmm' sound with each slow breath out, but this isn't really necessary unless you're meditating in the traditional Buddhist way.

Don't worry if you can't imagine this to start with – it comes with a little practice. Once it starts to happen, you'll know the feeling. All your thoughts become focused into the tunnel, all distractions sucked in, and your head becomes wonderfully uncluttered.

After a few minues of this, you can simply open your eyes and 'snap out of it'. If you're doing it right, you'll feel greatly refreshed.

Massage

Tense muscles knot into tender trigger spots. A wonderful way of releasing the spasm is to massage and stretch the muscles. Whilst yoga uses long, slow stretches along the line of action of the muscles, massage involves rhythmic pressure across their line of action.

The muscles most responsive to massage are those that are held rigid and static for most of the day – in particular, the muscles at the back of the head, neck, shoulders and down the back of the trunk. Massage of the feet is also wonderfully relaxing. Needless to say, you need someone else to do the masssage for you.

Lie face down, preferably after a warm bath, and preferably naked or nearly so. A few drops of an aromatic oil helps to smooth the action, and will also smell rather nice.

There are many different techniques that can be used. Some involve firm, steady kneading strokes with the flats of the hands, some deeper rotary movements with the heels of the hands or thumbs. Others employ the knuckles or fingertips. Still others employ rapid clapping or pounding movements. The important thing is not to touch too lightly because the slightest tickle will ruin everything. It's best to work systematically down the spine.

Yoga

The practice of yoga began in India some 3,000 years ago and it's only in the last few decades that it's really caught on in the Western world. Now yoga classes are among the most popular available, attracting a wide spectrum of people of both sexes and all ages.

Yoga in the fullest meaning of the word is a philosophical and practical discipline embracing the spiritual, moral, mental and physical fulfilment of the devotee. However, the more limited form that's most widely practised consists simply of a series of physical and mental exercises, postures or attitudes which relax the body and refresh the mind. The emphasis is on balance, muscle control and gentle stretching. The teaching usually also involves deep breathing and meditation.

Rhythmic activity

The physical benefits of rhythmic aerobic activities were described in the previous chapter. However, there's no doubt that most non-competitive rhythmic forms of exercise, such as skipping, running, dancing and swimming, are all great ways of releasing tension, providing you can find a hassle-free time and place for them.

Warm baths, soft music, sex – and other distractions

Wonderful ways of winding down. What more need be said?

SLEEP, DRIFTING SLEEP

We spend about a third of our lives asleep. But, far from being a waste of time, sleeping is a vital function of the body. During sleep, most of the brain is simply ticking over and the neurones' chemical batteries are recharged. It's also a time when the body's resources do most of the tissue repair.

Despite this shutdown, parts of the brain are very active during certain periods of sleep. These periods, characterised by rapid eye movements under the closed lids, are called REM sleep. Dreaming is intense at these times, and it's been shown that people who are deprived of REM sleep, wake up irritable and unrefreshed. Too much alcohol or some types of sleeping tablet will reduce REM sleep, which accounts in part for the poor quality of relaxation gained from such sleep. A further sleep in the afternoon is often far more refreshing.

People need different amounts of sleep and often the quality is more important than the quantity. Older people do not need to sleep as long, but find 'cat naps' through the day more refreshing.

Different countries also have customs with regard to sleep. In hot climates such as the Mediterranean, people may break from work in the afternoon and go to bed for a short 'siesta'. They then tend to work on into the evening and have a late evening meal – a very sensible routine.

Poor sleep patterns

About one person in ten has difficulty sleeping, and it's one of the commonest reasons for seeing the GP. Whether it be difficulty getting off to sleep, disturbed nights, poor quality sleep, or early waking, it's a form of insomnia. The result is all too likely to be daytime drowsiness, tetchiness, strained relationships, poor performance, difficulty coping, aches and pains, depression, and an increased risk of accidents.

It's a problem suffered by only about 5 per cent of under-thirty-year-olds – but as many as one in three of the over sixty-fives – especially women.

But why does it happen? And what can sufferers do about it?

What causes it?

The most common cause is worry – especially personal or family problems, work, or money. Sometimes it's simply worrying about the lack of sleep! An anxious state of mind prevents the brain's activating centre from 'switching off' – so that thoughts go round and round, and you find yourself constantly churning the same things over and over again.

Another common cause is physical discomfort or pain – anything from flatulence to arthritis, backache to breathlessness.

Noise is a frequent cause – perhaps the all-night party down the road, or your partner's snoring next to you.

It might be eating or drinking the wrong things too late at night – spicy foods, strong cheeses, coffee or tea – which contain stimulants. Or it might be too much alcohol – which may disturb your natural sleep pattern so that you wake up at 3 a.m. and can't get off again.

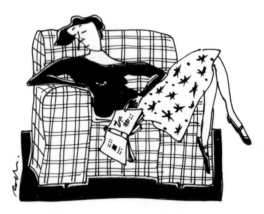

Too much catnapping in the daytime will disturb your sleep at night

Who's most susceptible?

Apart from these common causes, insomnia is more likely in women with premenstrual syndrome and in those going through the menopause. It's also a problem for older men with prostate trouble and a weak bladder. Shift workers are prone to insomnia, as are people with jet-lag. People who take cat-naps a lot during the day tend to have a poor night's sleep. But we are all more susceptible on some nights more than others simply because of natural rhythms in our brain chemistry.

What can be done to help?

First, don't worry if you're not getting your eight hours sleep a night. Research shows that, contrary to popular belief, most people don't need this much. Six hours of good quality sleep is about right, once you've got into the habit. And the older you are, the less sleep you'll need.

Get your bedtime routine right. Go through all the rituals to get yourself into a relaxed frame of mind. Have a nice warm bath followed by a cup of malt drink or cocoa, or camomile tea. Listen to some soothing music. Avoid alcohol late at night, and caffeine-containing drinks – and don't smoke within an hour of bedtime.

Try using an alarm clock – even if you don't have to get up early. It helps to train you into waking up at a particular time each morning, and this will reset your body-clock to make you naturally sleepy at bedtime.

If you're suffering from aches and pains, you may find that a firmer mattress or more pillows help to make you more comfortable, and less likely to lie awake.

Can the doctor help?

Apart from giving advice, your doctor may be able to find the underlying cause of your insomnia and deal with it. For example, all that may be needed is a painkiller or antidepressant medication.

Sleeping tablets can often break the vicious cycle of insomnia leading to daytime catnapping, leading to more insomnia. But the quality of sleep isn't very good, and there's often a problem with drowsiness next day. What's more, people can easily become psychologically dependent on them.

For these reasons, doctors are usually loath to prescribe sleeping tablets except in desperate cases – and even then only a short course to get the person over some crisis, such as bereavement.

Help yourself to a good night

1. Try to find out why you're not sleeping well. Is it pain, discomfort, noise, worry?

2. See if you can deal with it in some simple way. Eat earlier in the evening. Have a warm bath. Give yourself an extra blanket.

3. Avoid caffeine-containing drinks, such as coffee and tea, in the two hours before bedtime. Try a warm milky drink instead.

4. Avoid spicy or stimulating foods late at night. Avoid cigarettes. And, whilst a little alcohol may help you sleep, don't drink too much.

5. Avoid vigorous exercise late at night – apart from sex. Intercourse is a great way to relax the mind and body.

6. Don't read scary books or watch exciting videos just before bed.

7. If insomnia is causing you real problems, see your doctor.

DEPRESSION

We all get depressed from time to time. Disappointments, money worries, relationship problems, trouble at work, or the bitter blow of losing a loved one. Let's face it – for most of us there's plenty to be depressed about. But although we may tell ourselves we're feeling depressed, it's usually not depression in the true sense of the word.

What doctors call depression, or rather depressive illness, is more than simply feeling low, miserable and down-in-the-dumps. After all, it's perfectly normal and natural to feel fed up if things aren't going well. We sigh a lot – perhaps cry a lot – but we still carry on.

In most cases of true depression, this drive to carry on is lost. Apart from the emotional low, many other aspects of normal functioning may be affected – so many that carrying on in any meaningful way becomes increasingly difficult. Depression becomes a huge burden in itself, interfering with health – truly a depressive illness – as though being weighed down by a heavy blanket.

What are the other symptoms?

Disturbances of sleep, lack of self-confidence, changes of appetite, loss of interest in sex, slowness of thought, difficulty concentrating, poor memory, agitation or anxiety, irritability, unprovoked tearfulness, a sense of hopelessness, and of course in some cases suicidal thoughts. These are the symptoms most often involved in the illness – but most people with depression will only experience a few of these at any one time. They also tend to come and go to some extent.

Are there different types of depression?

Yes, although drawing a distinction isn't always easy. There are clearly people whose depression is an over-reaction to some loss, disappointment or bereavement. They can't shake off the misery, and they sink deeper and deeper into depression.

Another type descends on the sufferer for no apparent reason. They have no particular worries or anxieties – but they find themselves becoming more and more miserable. This type may be linked to hormonal or chemical changes in the body, affecting the mood centre in the brain.

There are well recognised versions of this latter type. For instance, SAD – seasonal affective disorder or 'winter blues' – affects many people during the dark gloomy days of winter. The depression that may follow viral illnesses, such as flu, is another example. Or the dreadfully heavy numbing feeling that some people experience after eating certain foods.

Many women suffer quite severe depression in the few days before their periods, or during the year or two around their menopause – and a substantial number suffer postnatal depression in the weeks or months after the birth of their baby.

Depression may also be linked to a chronic drinking problem and various diseases such as an under-active thyroid gland.

Suicidal thoughts

Many people get to the stage when they consider ending it all. Perhaps surprisingly, the danger time for this is not when they are in the deepest depths of depression, but when they have recovered sufficiently to have the determination to do something about it – even though that something is to do away with themselves.

What can be done to help?

Unfortunately some people find it hard to understand depression and there is a temptation to adopt the 'pull yourself together' attitude which invariably succeeds only in making things worse. Sympathy is what's needed.

In milder cases, particularly those triggered by a loss or disappointment, sharing the sufferer's problems by talking things over, offering a shoulder to cry on, and helping out in other ways can make all the difference. Keep emphasising the positive. Encourage the person to get out and about. Persuade him or her to take up a physical activity previously enjoyed. Try to keep the individual busy and engaged.

If the cloud refuses to lift, they may need to see their doctor, who can attempt to sort out what's at the root of the depression. It may be necessary for them to have a short course of anti-depressant therapy to reverse the downward spiral of despair. In some cases, the depressed person may be so ill that they need to be referred to see a specialist at the psychiatric outpatients department. The relatively few sufferers who are threatening suicide may need to be admitted to hospital until their depression has been successfully treated.

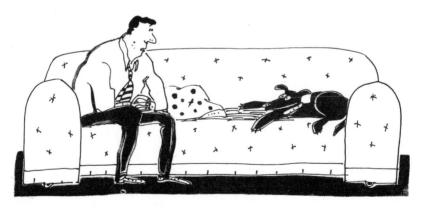

A problem shared is a problem halved

Self-help

1. If you are the sufferer, try to find someone to share your feelings with.

2. If a friend or loved one needs help and support, try to recognise the early symptoms of depression and, if necessary, encourage them to seek their doctor's advice.

3. If someone you know has expressed feelings about harming themselves or others in some way, try to persuade them to call a helpline such as the Samaritans or to see their doctor.

General practitioners are specially trained to recognise and treat depression. They are a natural source of help, especially if they have some knowledge of your circumstances. Treating depression is as much a part of their everyday work as treating high blood pressure, so don't feel you're wasting their time. And don't assume that you will automatically be put on some anti-depressant treatment. Talking about your feelings will be just as much a part of dealing with the problem. Many GPs also employ trained counsellors. It's surprising how much better you can feel by sharing your worries and problems with someone who is outside your immediate circle and who has no axe to grind other than helping you to feel better.

How life can get you down

Many events can have a powerful effect on our mood and in some cases lead to depression. Here are some of the most likely.

- Bereavement, particularly of a partner or child.
- Divorce or break-up of a relationship.
- Redundancy or loss of job.
- Moving home.
- Chronic or incurable physical illness.
- Misuse of alcohol

Men at risk

Perhaps surprisingly, it is younger men who are most likely to commit suicide. Being made redundant or losing a job is thought to be one of the main reasons. So too is the break-up of a relationship, perhaps divorce. Men it seems can't cope as well as women with such disasters, and they're not so good at sharing their problems. Another factor is alcohol – men are more likely to turn to drink and kill themselves under the influence.

Postnatal depression

At around three days after the birth of a baby, there is often a period of the 'baby blues'. It usually passes quickly but occasionally remains for weeks, months or longer. In severe cases, the depressed mother may be rendered incapable of coping with her everyday existence, including care of her baby or any other children in the family. Postnatal depression responds well to treatment from the doctor but must be recognised early as it can be confused with general tiredness and fatigue which is often the natural result of a new baby in the house.

COPING WITH LOSS

Most people underestimate the effects of bereavement. Often the bereaved person doesn't realise that the loss of interest in their job or family, constant pacing of the floor, spontaneous weeping or lack of appetite, are all normal and common manifestations of grieving.

People who are close to the bereaved person may also fail to understand its full effects, becoming unsympathetic, intolerant or impatient, especially after some weeks or months.

It is at this point that true friends are worth their weight in gold. To know when to leave the person alone and when to sit and listen, often to the same story over and over again without interruption, is a gift that few people have nowadays.

Thankfully, there are voluntary or professional agencies who specialise in this form of counselling and can be contacted through your GP. Nobody pretends that strangers can provide the same support as sympathetic friends or relatives, but they can often help to a person who has difficulty coming to terms with loss.

If you, or someone close to you, suffer a loss, remember:

- **Talk about it, even if it hurts.**
- **People have different ways of expressing grief, there is no 'normal way'.**
- **Don't be afraid to seek support from friends, relatives or your doctor.**
- **Allow yourself time to grieve, and try to avoid becoming reliant on drink or drugs, whether the latter are prescribed or not.**

STAGES OF GRIEF

1. *Denial:* 'It can't be true'. 'This can't have happened'.

2. *Anger:* 'Who's fault was it?' 'Why has it happened to me?'

3. *Guilt:* 'I should have done more'. 'If only I'd tried harder'.

4. *Acceptance:* 'What will be, will be'. 'It's happened, and that's that'.

5. *Coming to Terms:* 'Better make the best of things'. 'Got to get on with life'. 'Time will heal'.

ALCOHOL

Drink is an easy way to relax, a source of much pleasure and a great social lubricant. For most people in the developed world, life would be rather dreary without it.

The trouble, as we all know, is that it has a 'down side'. Apart from a long list of social problems linked to over-indulgence – from accidents to arson, and from marital bust-ups to pub punch-ups – there are several major, long-term health risks. Most people know that alcohol can lead to such disorders as cirrhosis of the liver, vitamin deficiency and loss of memory brought on by chronic heavy drinking. But not so many are aware of the link between excessive drinking and high blood pressure. In fact, over-indulgence in alcohol is about twice as common among hypertensive people as among those with normal blood pressure.

In fact, altogether, one in eight admissions to hospital is alcohol-related. This includes violence, traffic accidents and illness as a direct result of excessive drinking. There has been a rapid rise in alcohol-related admissions over the past ten years. This appears to have a direct correlation with the relative cost of alcohol, which is cheaper now, in real terms, than it has ever been.

Within limits

There are clear guidelines from most national expert bodies on the limits for 'sensible' drinking. In Britain, for instance, the Royal College of Physicians, together with a number of other eminent organisations, has recommended the following as sensible limits:

- **For men:**   21 units of alcohol a week.
- **For women:**   14 units of alcohol a week.

Now, these limits may strike you as somewhat spartan. After all, many women would find just two glasses of wine a day a touch mean. And a lot of men would consider half a pint of lager at lunchtime and a pint in the evening as virtually teetotal.

And yet, for some people, any more than this and the risks begin to rise.

What's a 'unit' of alcohol?

- Half a pint of *ordinary* beer, lager or cider

- A pub glass of table wine

- A small pub measure of sherry, vermouth or port

- A single pub measure of gin, whisky, vodka or other spirit

Remember these are pub measures. Drinks poured out at home tend to be rather more generous.

Drinking dangers

The statistics speak for themselves. There are about one million people in Britain whose lives and health have been seriously damaged by alcohol. Every year, over 28,000 people die before their time from alcohol-related illnesses. At least 1,000 young people are killed every year as a result of accidents or violence linked to alcohol. And drink is a common factor in at least half of all crimes committed against people or property.

There's no doubt that alcohol misuse of one form or another places a huge burden on society, both in terms of human misery and economic cost. In many cases the damage results from the occasional binge, drinking spree or simply a drink too many, but in a high proportion the root cause is 'alcoholism', or rather alcohol dependence – more commonly called a 'drink problem'.

What is alcohol dependence?

It's the need to drink even though the habit is making life difficult, either for the drinker or other people. Perhaps the person drinks too much each time, or too often, or at the wrong time, or in the wrong place. But the constant factor is the irresistible need for a drink.

The term 'alcoholic' is not used so much these days because it suggests that the drinker is somehow different from other people, with perhaps a biochemical susceptibility to alcohol. We now know this is a false distinction, and that any of us could become dependent on alcohol – needing to drink too much, too often.

But only a minority of dependent drinkers develop a real physical need to drink, with real withdrawal symptoms if they go without – rather like the craving for nicotine or heroin. Most are psychologically dependent on the habit – they need to indulge in the ritual of drinking or the carefree mental state it produces rather than to fend off the awful feeling of not having alcohol.

And what is problem drinking?

In the simplest terms, it's when someone's drinking causes problems, either for themselves or for someone else. So, for example, it might be night after night in the pub, making the person late for work in the mornings. Or the tipple or two too many at lunchtime – and falling asleep on the job in the afternoon. Or steady sipping throughout the day leading to rows and bust-ups in the evenings.

How does problem drinking start?

The important thing to realise is that there's no hard and fast dividing line between OK drinking and problem drinking – the one often merges into the other. Nor is there always a clear dependence on alcohol – some problem drinkers could give it up or cut down if they really wanted to.

But most people with a drinking problem either aren't aware of it, or refuse to admit to themselves that their drinking is beginning to get out of hand.

What are the warning signs?

Again there are no definite rules – but plenty of clues that things aren't quite right.

For example, does the person drink because they're bored, or unhappy, or stressed, or angry? Do they drink to feel better?

More importantly, does the person look forward to their next drink? Are they drinking faster than their friends? Do they need a drink before important events? Do they switch to doubles for no real reason?

Are other people noticing their drinking? Are they always the one to have a quick last drink? Are they spending too much on booze? Are they drinking more than they did a year ago?

Or, as the habit gets more of a grip ... Are they beginning to feel they may have a problem? Are they having trouble at work? Rows with family or friends? Are things not getting done? Bills not being paid? Are they drinking in the mornings? Do they have a secret supply of booze?

Of course, most problem drinkers won't be showing all these signs. But if someone you know has a few of them, it may mean that they need help.

What can be done to help?

The first thing is to talk it over with the person as carefully and sensitively as you can. If you push too hard they may react by clamming up and denying the whole thing. Try and get them to open up about themselves – their hopes and fears, their joys and sorrows – over a drink if necessary.

If they recognise that they have a drink problem, or at least might have the beginnings of, then they may be prepared to seek some help, or accept it if it's offered. This might be from their doctor, priest or other trusted person, or perhaps from one of several organisations who can advise and guide people who have problems linked to drink. Confidential helplines are available for anonymous counselling. Or, for those who prefer to meet others with similar problems, there are local groups where drinkers can share ways of coping and conquering their need for alcohol.

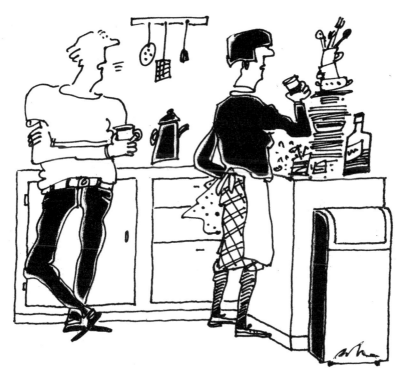

Never drink out of boredom

Self-help

1. If you think your drinking may be becoming too much of a habit, keep a diary of what you drink, when and why. Drinking is definitely harmful to

your health if it exceeds thirty-five units a week for a woman and fifty units for a man.

2. Try to find out what makes you want each drink. Is there some trigger you can avoid?

3. Try to cut down on alcoholic drinks. Have something non-alcoholic. Or choose a longer drink and make it really last.

4. Find other ways to relax and enjoy yourself. A visit to the leisure centre, a walk in the park, an evening class – anything to keep away from drink and drinkers.

Drink and driving

More people are seriously injured by drink-drivers in this country than are mugged or assaulted, and more are killed by drink-drivers than are murdered.

And yet all it takes to cause one of these awful statistics, or to become one, is just a few sips of alcohol too many.

Most people underestimate the effects of alcohol on their judgment of speed and distance, and accident proneness. You don't have to be drunk to be a killer. Startling though it may seem, even if you drink no more than the legal limit in Britain, your chances of an accident are doubled. And if you drink to the point of being pleasantly merry, your risk of an accident is *tenfold*.

How to change your drinking habits
- Eat before you drink.
- Try low alcohol drinks.
- Use mixers, avoid drinking neat spirits.
- Sip your drink, avoid the 'down in one' mentality.
- Have drink-free days, give your body a chance to recover.
- Try to avoid drinking alone at home.

Units of alcohol

Beers and Lagers	*Units*
1 pint of Export beer	2.5
1 can of Export beer	2
1 pint of ordinary beer or lager	2
1 can of ordinary beer or lager	1.5
1 pint of strong ale or lager	4
1 can of strong ale or lager	3
1 pint of extra-strong beer or lager	5
1 can of extra-strong beer or lager	4
Cider	
1 pint of cider	3
1 pint of strong cider	4
Spirits	
1 standard single measure (England)	1
1 standard single measure (Northern Ireland)	1.5
Table wine	
1 standard glass	1
Sherry/Vermouth/Port	
1 standard small measure	1

'Low alcohol' drinks
The levels of alcohol can vary enormously. Only if the label states
'alcohol free' can it be taken that there is virtually no alcohol present.

Now the Good News

Research has shown that your heart and arteries may actually benefit from a
couple of drinks each day. Red wine is probably the most valuable form and
may partly explain the low incidence of heart disease around the
Mediterranean. It would appear to inhibit the laying down of fats in the artery
walls. Also, acting as a mild diuretic, it helps the kidneys to function and may
lower blood pressure.

Unfortunately, the beneficial effects are rapidly lost once this small amount is
exceeded.

Cheers!

SMOKING

The easiest thing for a doctor to do is to tell someone to stop smoking. Conversely, the hardest thing for some smokers is to do just that. Many of them really enjoy their cigarettes. For some it's the only pleasure they have.

And yet, survey after survey shows that more and more smokers really want to give up. Or rather, they do and they don't. They would like to have given up, to be non-smokers. But they don't like the idea of going through the process – the 'cold turkey'.

If you're one of these 'floating smokers', hovering on the brink of stopping, here are some hints on how to go about it. It needn't be as traumatic as you might think.

First, remind yourself why

You know very well that smoking increases your risk of heart disease, chronic bronchitis and lung cancer. But you may not be aware that it's also linked to many other diseases, including cancer of the cervix, bladder, throat and pancreas. It triggers peptic ulcers and worsens arterial disease, including that caused by diabetes. It increases the risk of miscarriage and the problems associated with a low birthweight baby.

Is your child a nico-tiny?

You can make up your own mind about smoking. But are you forcing your baby or young child to smoke?

Watch your child's breathing. It's much faster than your own. This means that any smoke in the air is rapidly being inhaled by those brand-new pink lungs. Isn't it a shame to turn those dirty grey with the smoke from your cigarettes? There's no doubt that some forms of childhood lung disease, asthma in particular, is increased in this way. Children of smokers are also more likely to suffer from glue ear.

Apart from all this, smoking pollutes the air people have to breathe, smells awful, is a fire hazard and costs a lot of money.

How to Stop

The chances are you've tried giving up before – perhaps more times than you care to remember. But were you *really* determined to succeed? Did you have enough encouragement and support? Did you follow a method, or just throw yourself into it?

There's no question that nicotine is a highly addictive drug. Although it lacks the euphoric effects of heroin, its ability to 'hook' the user is not so very different. If cigarettes had been introduced on the streets today, they would have been banned immediately.

This means that many hardened smokers find it very difficult to give up. For them the anxiety and irritability – the 'cold turkey' – is too much to bear. The relief at finally capitulating, at having that much-craved-for cigarette, is overwhelming. It puts them back on the rails again. But it's a tragedy as far as their health is concerned, because these heavy smokers have most to gain from stopping.

The majority of smokers, thank goodness, aren't as physically dependent on nicotine as this, and giving up needn't be anywhere near so difficult. If you're a smoker you'll know how long you can go without a cigarette. You'll know that it depends on what you're doing, who you're with and where you are. You may even have found that, in some circumstances, you can go all day without a cigarette and not miss it.

Much of the smoking habit is just that – a habit. You've got used to doing it at particular times of the day or in particular places – perhaps with your morning coffee, or whenever you're on the phone, or if you're waiting somewhere, or in the car, or at the pub, or at home watching TV. In other words, you find yourself in 'trigger situations' and – ping! – a bell rings in your subconscious and you reach for the fags. Pure Pavlov.

So, to win at giving up smoking, you may have to overcome two hurdles, depending on what kind of a smoker you are. If nicotine is important to you, you'll have to shake off your physical and psychological dependence on it. And if you're locked into the ritual of smoking, you'll have to find ways of avoiding or breaking the triggers.

Steps to success

Here's a simple approach to giving up that covers both of these aspects and should suit nearly all smokers.

1. Make the decision and stick to it.

This is the absolutely crucial first step. Unless you're convinced you want to be a non-smoker, and that this time you're really going to make sure you succeed, you won't stand a chance. Rethink all the reasons for giving up. Write them down, and put them in priority order. Think how much better things will be when you're a non-smoker. Not 'if', but 'when'. Try to persuade your friend, partner or workmate to give up with you – you can do a lot to help each other win through.

2. Prepare to stop.

As with any battle, preparation is vital. Name a date to give up in a week or two's time – don't leave it any longer. It's no use saying you'll wait until the pressure's off a bit – it never will be. Pick as typical a day as possible.

Tell your friends and colleagues (especially the non-smokers) about your decision, and which day you'll be stopping. It will help reinforce your determination.

Cut down the number of cigarettes you smoke in the week beforehand. Miss out the less important ones. One trick is to put a rubber band round the packet so that you have to ask yourself each time – do I really need this one right now? Another trick is not to carry any lighter or matches so that you have to keep asking for a light.

3. The day you stop.

The moment you wake up, tell yourself you're now a non-smoker. You've done it. Make the mental leap. Convince yourself that, rather than being a smoker who's struggling to give up, you're a non-smoker who doesn't need to smoke and is not going to. True, you're only a beginner at non-smoking (or shall we say out of practice!), and you may have some difficulty to start with, but, basically, you're a natural non-smoker and you won't have any cigarettes in your mouth today. None. Not one.

Aim to just get through this one day without a cigarette. Don't contemplate tomorrow, the next week or two, or the rest of your life. Just take one day at a time.

Remove all lighters, ashtrays and other smoking paraphernalia from your presence. Carefully avoid your smoking trigger situations. For example, have an orange juice instead of coffee, a sandwich in the park instead of a pub lunch, chew sugar-free gum when you're on the phone. Find diversions and distractions. If you find yourself in a tough spot and desperate, try deep breathing.

4. Staying stopped.

Follow the same principles as for yesterday. Take one day at a time. Find new ways of avoiding triggers – non-fattening things to chew or munch, things to do with your hands, fresh-tasting drinks instead of coffee or tea, new places to go in your breaks.

If you're worried about putting on weight, surround yourself with low-calorie comforters – mineral water, low-cal drinks, sugar-free gum, fruit.

Keep on your guard. It's very tempting after a week or two, or a few months, to tell yourself that you've cracked it and you can now have just one little ciggie as a reward. Oh woe! The classic error.

Tips for success

- Heavier smokers should allow an extra three or four weeks cutting down before they give up completely.
- Hypnosis or acupuncture can certainly help some people to give up smoking.
- If you're particularly dependent on nicotine, try using nicotine gum, available from pharmacists without prescription. Nicotine skin patches are another method. They can double your chance of success.
- Save the money you would have spent on cigarettes and give yourself a real treat.

> When really tempted, try to imagine your lungs as a pair of very full ashtrays after a party. Perhaps not a million miles away from the truth.

Some questions answered

Q. How long will it take for the craving to stop?

A. This varies. Some people find they are free from craving within a few days, for others it can take weeks.

Q. Could I not have just the occasional puff?

A. The answer is an emphatic 'NO'. It's the slippery slope back to smoking.

Q. Will I put on weight?

A. Not necessarily, although some people do. Remember that weight gain after giving up smoking is usually temporary, perhaps lasting two or three weeks whilst the metabolism readjusts to the absence of nicotine. Then, as long as you're not consuming more calories, you should start to shed it again.

Q. How long will it take to recover from the harm of cigarettes?

A. A great deal depends upon what harm you have done already. You will immediately be free from the carbon monoxide and other poisons. Within days your breath will be fresher and your teeth cleaner. Your breathing and some circulation problems will resolve within weeks. The risk of heart disease starts to reduce very quickly. That of lung cancer takes longer. But from the day you give up, your health prospects will improve – and so will those of your young children.

- Early death from tobacco is common. Around 2,000 people in the UK do it every week. During the six years of the Second World War a quarter of a million UK people were killed. In the past five years, tobacco has killed about twice that number.

- In the UK tobacco kills about four times as many people as the total killed by drink, drugs, murder, suicide, road accidents, rail accidents, air accidents, poisoning, drowning, fires, falls, snakes, lightning and every other known form of accidental death all put together.

Don't give up giving up!

Sadly, some smokers, no matter how convinced they are about the dangers of smoking, and how much they say they want to give up, simply can't manage to kick the habit.

Yet thousands do succeed, despite these difficulties. And you can too. The stumbling block is all in the mind. If you've tried to give up, only to have failed miserably, don't worry, you're in good company. Just try again – but really go for it this time. Most people will make more than one attempt before eventually winning

DRUGS

All kinds of misconceptions surround the subject of drug abuse. The stereotypical drug addict is only the tip of the iceberg when we look more carefully at the problem. For example, apart from alcohol, tobacco and caffeine, which are far and away the most widely used drugs, persistent dependence on prescribed tranquillisers, antidepressants and sleeping tablets is a major cause for concern.

Such is the fear, ignorance and prejudice surrounding the whole question of drugs that it's seldom realised that there's more than one way of taking drugs and that, not only is there a wide range of drugs with different effects, but that these will differ between individuals.

- **Some drugs are used in more unsafe ways than others. Injection is almost always more hazardous than sniffing or smoking them.**
- **People have different reasons for drug taking and the things which will help them stop will also be varied. It is impossible to generalise about drugs or drug users.**
- **Advice and practical help is variable across the country. Where you live can influence not only your exposure to illegal drugs, but also the support available to help you give them up.**

Just a passing phase?

For various reasons, each age group is more likely to use certain drugs or substances than others. Solvent abuse is most popular in the early teens, or even younger – the substances being 'borrowed' from around the home. Most users of ecstasy, acid and crack are in their late teens, and take these drugs to heighten their excitement at raves and parties. Cannabis and cocaine users tend to be rather older and are into the mind-bending effects on aesthetic perception. Users who inject drugs, such as heroin, need the 'hit' in order to feel well. Their habit is expensive and they are mainly in their twenties.

Do you keep on taking the tablets?

Dependence on drugs prescribed by your doctor can creep up on you. Not being able to sleep during a particularly stressful episode in life, and the consequent use of sleeping tablets can, if not carefully watched, go on to become an addiction. Tranquillisers too can be addictive. Even painkillers, such as aspirin, although not physically habit-forming, can be the cause of psychological dependence.

So too can laxatives!

Which drug? – a brief guide

Solvents
- Substances most likely to be experimented with by young people after first trying alcohol and tobacco.
- Includes aerosol sprays, butane gas, glues, paint thinners, type-correcting fluids and even petrol.
- Can cause respiratory arrest and chronic lung conditions.

Cannabis
- Most commonly used illegal drug.
- Wide variation in effect.
- Causes relaxation, talkativeness and altered perception, especially to time, space, music and mood.
- Little evidence of immediate harmful effects but the intoxication, like alcohol, may cause accidental harm.
- Often mixed with tobacco, which may cause the respiratory and other problems associated with that substance.
- No evidence that it leads to so called 'hard drugs' such as heroin.

Amphetamine

- The most widely used stimulant.
- Powder usually sniffed or injected.
- Single dose will last about three hours.
- Produces a state of alertness and heightened feeling of confidence.
- Exhaustion and confusion if used continually.
- Tolerance and the need for increasingly higher doses sets in rapidly.
- Can lead to paranoia and personality disturbance.
- Can affect the rhythm of the heart with fatal consequences.

Cocaine and Crack

- Powerful stimulants similar to amphetamines.
- Can be injected, sniffed or smoked (crack).
- Expensive and short-lived effects.
- Can cause all the problems of amphetamines along with respiratory disorders and chest pain.

Ecstasy

- Mixed stimulant with a delayed effect of around twenty minutes.
- Heightened perception of colours and sounds.
- Higher doses produces amphetamine effects.
- Deaths from cardiac arrest have occurred.

Acid (LSD) and Magic Mushrooms

- Not addictive.
- No known physical effects.
- Strongly psychedelic, altering perception, especially visual images and colours.
- Paranoia is a common side-effect.
- Nightmares which continue while awake are common.
- Flashbacks can recur for months afterwards.

Heroin

- Can be injected, sniffed or smoked.
- Produces a sense of warm and pleasant drowsiness. Novices may experience immediate nausea and vomiting.
- Strongly physically addictive. Lack of the drug causes a very unpleasant withdrawal illness.

- Many addicts take part in 'normal life' but only with the assistance of the drug. Finding the money to feed the addiction can lead to destitution or crime.
- Biggest danger is from injection, particularly when sharing needles. This can lead to HIV or hepatitis infection, thrombosis or gangrene.

Help for a drug problem

Your GP will always give confidential advice and help, but you can also find specialist helplines, support organisations and clinics listed in the phone book.

A HEALTHY LOVE LIFE

YOUR SEXUALITY

Sex is inescapable these days. It's hyped everywhere – papers, magazines, TV, radio and the cinema. Sex makes the world go round. Adverts flaunt it, selling anything from ice-cream to electric drills. Rock music throbs to it. Even children's TV is seething with a sanitised version of it.

Expectations of sex are high. We all believe so much in it, with or without love. And yet we're so ambivalent about it. We know it can be great. We also know it can be disastrous. And sometimes very confusing.

We think we understand quite a lot about sex – and yet there may be much we can't really fathom: about other people's sexuality and what drives it; about how love and sex can work with each other, or against each other; perhaps even about our own feelings about sex, our own sexuality. Small wonder that many of us have trouble enjoying a healthy love life.

Problems with sexuality

To admit to a problem with sexuality may not be easy – even just to oneself. Despite all the exposure, it's still an embarrassing subject. Part of the reason is that everyone has some reason to doubt, question or be concerned over their personal sexuality. Media hype certainly doesn't help by creating stereo-types which are impossible to live up to and can leave many with a feeling of inadequacy.

Many people worry whether their sexuality is normal, despite the fact that beyond what the media tell us, there is no definition of sexual normality. We have various religious concepts but even these vary between religions.

Homosexuality and bisexuality

While most of us are in no doubt, from adolescence, that we are strongly attracted to one sex or the other, some of us are confused about some of the feelings we experience, and it is not uncommon to discover after years of heterosexuality and even marriage that you also have feelings for your own sex.

Some people try to deny their attraction and actively seek partners of the opposite sex to prove to themselves and others that they aren't gay. Others 'come out' and accept their orientation. Practising gay sex still has a social stigma in some societies and is proscribed by law in others. Fortunately, prejudice against gay people is decreasing, especially in larger towns and cities with active gay communities.

Victorian blindness

Queen Victoria refused to accept the concept of female homosexuality and thus lesbianism was never made illegal or even submitted to the same medical category as was male homosexuality. Indeed, in Britain, gay men were still being subjected to electric shock therapy as recently as the 1970s. Male homosexuality was considered an 'illness' which needed to be 'cured'.

'I married my husband because he was the nicest man I'd ever met. Sex came with the marriage and it was the proverbial closing of the eyes and letting my mind wander. I never really enjoyed myself. Then one day I met Sara. I didn't realise I fancied her until she kissed me one night. It was wonderful. I just thought 'This is it'.'

'I'm a man who knows what's attractive and sexy in a woman, and I don't have any fear of women's sexuality. But I can also spot the same sexiness in a man. Very much so. That's what really turns me on.'

'I certainly don't think I'm missing out on anything being gay. I have no desire to have children or change my lifestyle. But I would like a long-term relationship with someone I love. And I'd like people to have a more liberal attitude towards gay men.'

'I used to think bisexual people were monsters with two heads. Since I've discovered I'm bisexual myself, I've had to change my view. I think there's a bit of bisexuality in everybody – some feelings towards both sexes. It's just a question of which ones are stronger at the time.'

'I've had relationships with men and women, and both have been great. At the moment I'm with a heterosexual man. I told him the night we met that I was bisexual. He was gobsmacked, but soon accepted me. We've had a good monogamous time together up to now, but I'm reluctant to close off the possibility of ever being with a woman again.'

'We decided on celibacy. And it's fine for both of us. Sometimes a favourite piece of music will remind me of when we used to have sex. But celibacy is like giving up smoking – you soon get used to it, and then wonder why you bothered about it so much before.'

Libido low?

Most worries about a lack of libido stem from an inappropriate expectation of sexual desire fuelled by images from the media. Libido and the need for sex vary among people as much as shoe size, and within the same person as much as the weather. Stress, time of the month, state of health, mood, past history – all have an effect on libido. And for many people, sex in any of its manifestations simply isn't what turns them on. That's OK – that's not abnormal.

Related to this is difficulty in reaching a climax, particularly for women. Approximately 40 per cent of women in a sexual partnership will achieve orgasm only occasionally, while fifteen per cent may never climax at all.

Sex therapy

Whilst most people would quite happily consult a doctor about their bodies, or a dentist about their teeth, few would contemplate consulting a counsellor or sex therapist about their sex problem. Yet sex is one of the most important things to many people, and these professionals are experts who can help.

Finding the underlying causes of any problems and rectifying them can dramatically improve relationships. For example, being taught how to use fantasies and sexual experimentation to improve your sex life, or being reassured that it isn't necessary always to reach a climax, which is often the cause of resentment and attempts to fake it.

Negative incidents can spoil things later on. Expecting too much can lead to disappointment, then worry. Failing to attain an erection can be interpreted by one partner as a lack of their attractiveness, while in the other as a sign of decreasing virility. A cycle of worry enters the relationship which causes even more stress and difficulty.

Sharing thoughts and feelings

Sex can be most enjoyable and fulfilling for both partners if you each know what you want and don't want from the relationship, you share your feelings, and you both understand that most problems stem from preconceived notions that remain hidden. Bringing them out and exploring ways round them can be both an exciting and loving experience.

If you have not been in the habit of talking about sex together, but performing in silence, you may find it easier to start talking out of bed – over a meal, doing the washing up, listening to music. When conversations like this become easy and natural, you should find that understanding each other in bed is much better.

Adding more spice

Even if a couple have been together for many years, there may be a lack of communication about what each would love their partner to do during their lovemaking. Sharing thoughts and feelings will help them discover mutual new pleasures. Making love in different ways, in different positions, at different times, in different places. It's surprising how many couples can revitalise their relationship in this simple way.

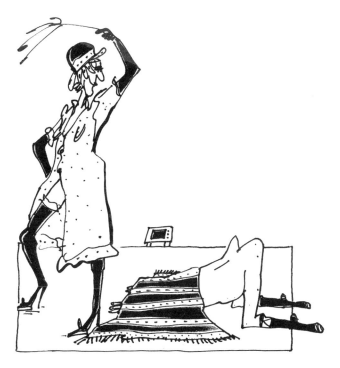

Experimentation can work wonders with a jaded sex life

A little of what he wants...
- appreciative and encouraging comments
- genuine enthusiasm
- uninhibited expressions of pleasure – sighs and gasps
- willingness to experiment
- gentle caresses, firm squeezes and bites – in the right places!

A little of what she wants...
- expressions of love and affection
- being made to feel special
- being told she's sexy
- enough foreplay
- gentle caresses, firm squeezes, hugs and kisses – also in the right places.

Saying no

Feeling OK about saying no when you want to is as important as feeling OK about saying yes. We all have the right to say no, and providing we do so in a sensitive, caring and responsible way, it should not be interpreted as a lack of love, affection or sexual desire for our partner.

Unfortunately, many male attitudes towards women, for instance, stem from a chauvinistic belief that women should always want sex, preferably when they themselves do. All too often a woman who refuses sex is dubbed as frigid. Not only grossly unfair – but wrong.

Privacy and peace

Distractions whilst lovemaking don't exactly help matters. Having the kids looked after by someone else for a couple of nights can do wonders for a jaded love life, and can produce the best sleep in years. Similarly, taking the phone off the hook can have a wonderfully tonic effect too.

A few intimate problems

Q. My sex life was always fairly lively. But since I've been married my enjoyment of sex has slowly but surely dwindled and is now practically non-existent. Even though my husband and I love each other dearly, we have horrid bedtime sulks. Please do you have any advice?

A. For women in particular, the sex-drive is a complex, mysterious and often delicate thing. Many factors could be turning you off sex. For example, it could be a change in your body chemistry – perhaps you've recently come off the Pill or switched to a different brand. Or your attitude may have changed – perhaps now you're married sex has become too predictable and even boring. Perhaps stress is playing a part.

Whatever the reason, guilt and resentment soon set in, making the problem much worse. The first step in tackling it is to talk it over together rather than just avoiding it. You may find that some simple change in the way you relate to each other brings a real improvement. Failing that, there are several popular paperbacks on the subject. Or you could seek help from a counselling organisation (see the phone book).

Q. I love my partner very much and greatly enjoy sex with him, but I can't reach a climax. What's going wrong?

A. *Most women have experienced this problem. Indeed, about one in seven have never had an orgasm, even though they enjoy sex. A common cause is anxiety – often about orgasm itself, about trying to come together, or about whether you'll be able to come at all. The temptation is to fake it – and that in itself causes more anxiety.*

The only way to break this vicious circle is by understanding that enjoyment of sex, for each of you, doesn't all hinge on your being able to come. You don't have to stage an Oscar-winning portrayal of ultimate ecstasy. And he mustn't feel that you have to hit the jackpot every time. So, be frank and honest with him and talk things over together. If he's remotely caring he'll help you to relax and just let things happen at their own pace and in their own time. This lets you explore other positions and ways of caressing each other that may give you the stimulation you need.

Q. My boyfriend and I have a terrific sex life. He's a great lover and I almost always have a climax. But it only happens when he strokes my clitoris and not by intercourse. Is this abnormal?

A. *No. It's the same for very many women. Some need deep vaginal penetration, some need pressure on the so-called 'G–spot' on the front wall of the vagina, and some, like you, need clitoral stimulation. If whatever you're doing is giving you both a good time, stop worrying about it and just carry on.*

Q. I am a forty-seven year-old male, and for nearly a year now I've been unable to get a proper erection. This is frustrating for both of us and I wonder whether there's anything I or my partner could do or take to get it back again.

A. *As many as one man in ten suffers from impotence. About half of them have a psychological reason for it – perhaps stress, depression or a particular anxiety – which is sapping their sex-drive but is often only temporary. Others have a physical cause – perhaps the side-effect of medication or a complication of diabetes.*

All men experience impotence at some time in their lives, but anxiety can make matters worse. So, take the pressure off yourself for a while by being content just to cuddle. Then, after a few weeks, ask your partner very gradually to begin to stroke and massage you again, all over, but avoiding your genital area — it's important not to think about what's happening there. Hopefully, in time, normal service will be resumed. If there's a physical cause for your difficulty, you will need advice and treatment from your doctor.

Q. I'm twenty and afraid to have sex with my present boyfriend. The problem is his erect penis is extremely large and I worry that penetration to this extent will damage me internally. I'd be grateful for your advice.

A. *You needn't fear dire consequences! The vagina is a very resilient organ. Not only does it expand in diameter during sex, it also becomes longer. Providing you don't feel pain when he's thrusting into you, no harm will be done.*

If you do experience discomfort, this may be because his penis is pushing against a tender part of your cervix, or because anxiety is making you too dry. Try putting a pillow between you both to prevent penetration from being too deep, and if necessary use a vaginal lubricant from the chemist.

Q. I feel attracted to another woman. Does this mean I'm bisexual, and should I tell my husband?

A. *If your feelings about the other woman amount to more than emotional intimacy together with a desire to be with her, this doesn't necessarily mean you're bisexual. It may reflect a need for a relationship that's physically unthreatening or 'neutral'. Or it may be just a passing fad or fancy.*

But if it's likely to be a lasting desire, then it's best to be open and honest about it with your husband, even though the shock is likely to shake your relationship with him severely — at least to start with. If he's a truly loving husband, he'll accept you the way you are. He'll also know how difficult it will have been for you to pluck up the courage to come clean about it — and he will respect you for that. He will also appreciate that you want to share your innermost feelings with him.

Q. I really enjoy pleasuring myself, but I feel so guilty about it. Can it harm me physically or emotionally?

A. Masturbation itself isn't harmful – but the guilt certainly may be. Most men and women masturbate from puberty onwards, with varying frequency, often within happy and fulfilling sexual relationships. Masturbation offers an opportunity to explore what works for you sexually. The fact that it's based on sexual fantasy need not detract from 'the real thing' when it happens. Indeed it may even enhance the real thing – and often does. Sexual fantasy is a normal part of healthy and fulfilling lovemaking.

Q. I want sex all the time – much more often than my partner does. Is this normal and healthy in a woman?

A. Usually a woman's sex-drive varies throughout her monthly cycle. The sexiest time for most is in the week after a period. Less often it's around the time of ovulation (about mid-way between each period) – also the most fertile time. Surprisingly, many women want sex most during a period. The Pill may increase, or decrease, the sex-drive. Despite all this, it's not unusual, nor unhealthy, to want sex all the time – many women would love to feel like this. It only becomes a problem if you can't satisfy the desire, either by lovemaking with a partner, or by pleasuring yourself. Most women in this situation find ways of coping, perhaps by channelling their energy into other interests or activities. But sexual frustration can lead to difficult or embarrassing situations, and some women may need help from a qualified counsellor or therapist.

SAFER SEX

Despite the existence of sexually transmitted (venereal) diseases like gonorrhoea and syphilis since humans first huddled together under a sabre-toothed tiger-skin, until the AIDS epidemic struck in the mid-eighties there was very little advice on safer sex to be found in the media, in schools, or anywhere other than well-thumbed library books on sex and curly eared leaflets at the doctor's.

These days, anybody embarking on a new relationship – whether a casual fling or the 'real thing' – is all too aware of the need to practise safer sex. Not only is it crucial for protection against HIV and sexually transmitted diseases, but it is also a means of contraception. Perhaps surprisingly, it has the added benefit in helping to pave the way to a more open and satisfying sex life.

For one thing, since the HIV risk, sex has gone public. It's come out of the closet and is now discussed so openly that there's much less chance of feeling embarrassed about expressing your feelings and desires, your likes and dislikes. Buying, carrying and using condoms is acceptable for women as well as men.

Using condoms

Always use a condom for vaginal and oral sex with anyone you're not absolutely sure about – which is pretty well everyone apart from a long-term totally faithful partner. There are lots of shapes, sizes and even flavours to choose from. For anal sex, a condom is mandatory every time – use the thicker type, well lubricated.

Putting one on may take some practice but, once you have the knack, it needn't be a passion killer. Indeed, many men enjoy the sensation of their partner stroking their penis and rolling a condom on it. The sense of security is also conducive to more relaxed lovemaking.

Putting on a condom can be fun if it's part of foreplay when she slips it on him. A few tips...

- **make sure it's new and hasn't passed its expiry date. Condoms can perish**
- **take care not to tear it with fingernails or jewellery**
- **use finger and thumb to press the air out of the teat at the end *before putting it on***
- **roll it gently over the erect penis, making sure you start it the right way round**
- **afterwards, he should hold the rim as he withdraws to avoid spillage**

HIV and AIDS

HIV is a virus which attacks your immune system and can eventually cause AIDS or related illnesses. AIDS is a deficiency of the immune system which interferes with your ability to fight off infections. With treatment, AIDS can sometimes be controlled but cannot at present be cured. Nor is there a vaccine. AIDS is nearly always fatal.

HIV is passed from person to person by the exchange of infected blood and other body fluids such as semen, saliva and vaginal secretions. Unprotected sex and the sharing of injection needles or syringes are the commonest ways of catching or passing on the virus. A mother can pass the virus to her baby, either in the womb, during birth or through breastmilk. Other possible ways are through contaminated equipment when having a tattoo, acupuncture, ear-piercing or electrolysis. In some countries, HIV can be caught from contaminated blood transfusions.

HIV infection doesn't usually cause any noticeable symptoms until it leads to disease some years later. The only way to be sure is by having the HIV test on a sample of your blood.

Other STDs

Anyone who's sexually active can catch a sexually transmitted disease – even 100 per cent monogamous couples may pass thrush, herpes or genital warts to each other. So you shouldn't feel embarrassed or guilty if you get one. The important thing is to seek proper medical help straight away.

Safer sex (or celibacy) is the best protection. You can buy books on sexual health if you want more information, but here are the main symptoms to watch out for:

- **Unusual discharge from the penis or vagina**
- **pain or stinging when you urinate**
- **soreness or irritation of the genital area**
- **unusual lumps or bumps down below.**

Some STDs cause no symptoms in the woman until the fallopian tubes are damaged and she has difficulty conceiving. If you or your partner have any of these it's important to make an appointment with a GUM (genito-urinary medicine) clinic straight away. The service is free on the NHS and no doctor's letter is needed. The number should be in the phone book under 'Genito-urinary Medicine' (or 'GUM'), 'Sexually Transmitted Diseases' ('STD'), or 'Venereal Diseases' ('VD'). Or see your own GP.

More people are discovering that sex can be just as enjoyable without penetration.

Here are a few suggestions to try:

- caressing, pressing, and tickling each other by hand or foot in the most intimate places
- soaping each other in the shower or bath
- massage with talc or aromatic oil
- nuzzling
- kissing, sucking and licking – but *not* the penis without a condom nor the vagina without a dental dam
- using a vibrator – but if you share it, put a condom on it
- dancing and cavorting
- fantasy and role playing

CONTRACEPTION

Times have changed from when women used to cut the end off a lemon and use it as a crude form of diaphragm cap. Not only was it a fairly hit and miss process, it probably made both partners' eyes water.

Nowadays, the choice of rather more acceptable and effective contraceptive methods can be quite bewildering, and there are many factors which have to be taken into account when deciding which to opt for. Religious belief, age, sex, and lifestyle are the most obvious. Your GP or local family planning clinic can advise you. There are also national organisations and telephone helplines.

Natural methods

Some couples, for various reasons, can't use the usual forms of contraception. Instead they must rely on either avoiding intercourse altogether or on the so-called 'rhythm method' – avoiding those days around the time of ovulation (egg release) during the menstrual cycle when the woman is fertile. Working out this 'safe' time requires some skill and practice.

Emergency contraception

If you have had sex without using any method of contraception, or you think it might have failed for any reason, there are two emergency methods which can be used. Both are free, but you'll need to see a doctor, family planning clinic or hospital accident and emergency department quickly.

- the 'morning after pill' – actually two special doses of a hormone pill which must be started within three days (72 hours) of unprotected sex. The sooner the better.
- fitting an IUD (the 'coil') – this must be done within five days. Again, the sooner the better.

Reliability of contraceptive methods

Diaphragm or cap with spermicide	Natural methods	Sponge	
❏ With careful use 2 women in 100 will get pregnant in a year. ❏ With less careful use 2 to 15 women in 100 will get pregnant in a year.	❏ With careful use 2 women in 100 will get pregnant in a year. ❏ With less careful use 2 to 20 women in 100 will get pregnant in a year.	❏ With careful use 9 women in 100 will get pregnant in a year. ❏ With less careful use 9 to 25 women in 100 will get pregnant in a year.	How reliable is it?
❏ A flexible rubber device, used with spermicide, is put into the vagina to cover the cervix and must stay in for at least six hours after sex. ❏ Must be specifically fitted to make sure it is the right size.	❏ A woman keeps a daily record of her body temperature, changes in cervical mucus and other signs of ovulation. These tell her when she is most fertile and should avoid sex or use a barrier method (for example, condom or diaphragm).	❏ A soft round sponge containing spermicide is put into the vagina before sex to cover the cervix. ❏ Must stay in for 6 hours after sex.	How it works
❏ Can be put in any time before sex (if more than three hours before, extra spermicide is needed). ❏ May protect against cancer of the cervix and some sexually transmitted diseases. ❏ There are a variety of types to choose from.	❏ No side effects. ❏ No mechanical devices or hormones are used. ❏ Knowing when the woman is fertile means pregnancy can be planned. ❏ Gives a woman a greater awareness of her body.	❏ Works for 24 hours after insertion. ❏ You can have sex more than once without using extra spermicide. ❏ Suitable for those with reduced fertility – near menopause or breastfeeding. ❏ Can be bought at a pharmacy.	Advantages
❏ Putting it in can interrupt sex. ❏ Extra spermicide is needed if you have sex again. ❏ Fitting should be checked every twelve months and if you gain or lose more than 3kg (7lbs), or have a baby, miscarriage or abortion.	❏ Women with irregular periods, after childbirth and around the menopause may find this method difficult. ❏ Daily record keeping needed. ❏ May involve avoiding sex at some times of the month unless an extra method is used.	❏ Expensive and unreliable. ❏ Not available from all family planning clinics. ❏ Should not be used during a period. ❏ Some people are sensitive to spermicide.	Disadvantages
❏ Some people are sensitive to spermicide. ❏ Cystitis can be a problem for some diaphragm users. Changing to a slightly smaller or softer rimmed diaphragm or cap may help. ❏ Do not leave in for more than thirty hours.	❏ Method should be learnt from a specially trained teacher and some charge a fee. ❏ Some people use a condom or diaphragm during the fertile time rather than avoid penetrative sex.	❏ Do not leave in for more then 30 hours. ❏ No fitting is required as one size fits all.	Comments

Female sterilisation	Male sterilisation (vasectomy)	Combined pill	
❏ The failure rate can be 1 to 3 in 1000 depending on the method used.	❏ The failure rate is about 1 in 1000.	❏ With careful use less than 1 woman in 100 will get pregnant in a year. ❏ With less careful use 3 or more women will get pregnant in a year.	How reliable is it?
❏ A permanent method in which the fallopian tubes are cut or blocked so the eggs cannot travel down them to meet sperm.	❏ A permanent method in which the tubes carrying the sperm are cut, so sperm are not present in the semen that is ejaculated when a man 'comes'.	❏ Contains two hormones – oestrogen and progestogen – which stop a woman releasing an egg each month (ovulation).	How it works
❏ Very effective. ❏ Permanent. ❏ Is effective immediately after the operation.	❏ Very effective. ❏ Permanent. ❏ Operation takes 10–15 minutes and can be done at a doctor's surgery or clinic.	❏ Does not interrupt sex. ❏ Often reduces bleeding, period pain and pre-menstrual tension. ❏ Protects against cancer of the ovary and womb and some pelvic infections. ❏ Suitable for healthy non-smokers up to the menopause.	Advantages
❏ Rarely the tubes rejoin and the woman is fertile again.	❏ It usually takes a few months for all the sperm to disappear from the semen. ❏ Contraception must be used during this time until there are two negative sperm tests. ❏ Rarely the tubes rejoin and the man is fertile again.	❏ May not be suitable for some women. A full medical history should be taken. ❏ May be temporary minor side-effects. ❏ Not suitable for smokers over 35 or for women who are breastfeeding.	Disadvantages
❏ This is a permanent method and should not be chosen if in any doubt. ❏ Counselling is important. ❏ Time in hospital varies from one to three days depending on the type of operation. ❏ A few days rest needed afterwards.	❏ This is a permanent method and should not be chosen if in any doubt. ❏ Counselling is important. ❏ Likely to be bruising and some discomfort for a short time after the operation. ❏ A few days rest needed afterwards.	❏ Not reliable if taken over 12 hours late or after vomiting or severe diarrhoea, unless an extra method is used. ❏ Some drugs may stop the Pill working – a doctor or pharmacist can advise. ❏ Pill users should try not to smoke.	Comments

Progestogen-only pill	Injectable contraceptive	IUD	
❏ With careful use 1 woman in 100 will get pregnant in a year. ❏ With less careful use 4 or more women in 100 will get pregnant in a year.	❏ Less than 1 woman in 100 will get pregnant in a year.	❏ Less than 1 to 2 women in 100 will get pregnant in a year.	How reliable is it?
❏ The hormone progestogen, taken at the same time each day, causes changes making it difficult for sperm to enter the womb or for the womb to accept a fertilised egg. In some women it prevents ovulation.	❏ An injection releases the hormone progestogen very slowly into the body which stops ovulation.	❏ A small plastic and copper device is put into the womb. It prevents sperm from meeting the egg or may prevent an egg from settling in the womb.	How it works
❏ Does not interrupt sex. ❏ Useful for older women who smoke and women who cannot use the combined pill. ❏ Can be used when breastfeeding.	❏ Does not interrupt sex. ❏ An injection lasts for two months or three months, depending on the type used. ❏ May protect against cancer of the womb.	❏ Does not interrupt sex. ❏ Works as soon as it is put in. ❏ Can stay in for a minimum of five years.	Advantages
❏ May be temporary minor side-effects. ❏ Periods may be irregular, with some bleeding in between or be missed. ❏ May be less effective in women who weigh over 70kg (11 stone).	❏ Periods often become irregular or stop. Regular periods and fertility may take a year or more to return after stopping the injections. ❏ Some women gain weight.	❏ Periods may be heavier or longer and more painful. ❏ Unsuitable for women who have heavy and painful periods. ❏ Not a first choice for women who are not in a mutually faithful relationship because of the risk of pelvic infection.	Disadvantages
❏ Not reliable if taken over three hours late or after vomiting or severe diarrhoea, unless an extra method is used. ❏ Some drugs may stop the Pill working – a doctor or pharmacist can advise.	❏ The injection works for either two or three months. It cannot be removed from the body so any unwanted effects may continue during this time.	❏ Usually changed every 5 years. If fitted after the age of 40 can stay in until the menopause. ❏ Women are taught to check the IUD by feeling the threads high in the vagina.	Comments

Male condom	Female condom	
❏ With careful use 2 women in 100 will get pregnant in a year.. ❏ With less careful use 2 to 15 women in 100 will get pregnant in a year.	❏ There have been no large-scale studies to show this, but research suggests it should be as effective as the male condom.	How reliable is it?
❏ Made of very thin rubber it is put over the erect penis and prevents sperm from entering the woman's vagina.	❏ A soft polyurethane sheath lines the vagina and the area just outside, and prevents sperm from entering the vagina.	How it works
❏ Free from family planning clinics and also sold widely. ❏ May protect both partners from sexually transmitted diseases, including HIV. ❏ May protect against cancer of the cervix. ❏ Man can take responsibility for contraception.	❏ Can be put in any time before sex. ❏ May protect both partners from sexually transmitted diseases, including HIV. ❏ May protect against cancer of the cervix. ❏ Oil based products can be used with female condoms.	Advantages
❏ Putting it on can interrupt sex. ❏ May slip off or split if not used correctly. ❏ Man needs to withdraw as soon as he has ejaculated and be careful not to spill any semen.	❏ Putting it in can interrupt sex. ❏ Need to make sure the man's penis enters the condom and not between the vagina and the condom. ❏ May slip. ❏ Expensive to buy.	Disadvantages
❏ Use a new condom each time. ❏ Must be put on before the penis touches the woman's vagina. ❏ Use a condom with a BSI Kitemark on the pack and check expiry date. ❏ Oil based products, such as body oils, should not be used with male condoms as they damage them.	❏ Use a new condom each time and follow the instructions carefully. ❏ BSI Kitemark for female condoms not yet available. ❏ Sold widely and is free at some family planning clinics.	Comments

(Based on Family Planning Association research)

MAINLY FOR WOMEN

So far, most of what we have considered about healthy living applies equally to either sex. But in this section we look at aspects which are of particular concern to women. How you, as a woman, can help to maintain your mental and physical well-being despite such bodily disruptions as periods, pregnancy and the menopause. And how you can monitor the health of your breasts and cervix.

PERIOD PROBLEMS

The average age for menstruation to start is thirteen (varying between about ten and eighteen), and the average age for the menopause is about fifty (varying between about forty-five and fifty-five).

The average length of the menstrual cycle is twenty-eight days (varying between about twenty-three and thirty-three) but is commonly quite irregular. With each cycle, the period starts on average fourteen days after ovulation (egg release). This tends to be true even with irregular periods, which implies that irregular periods usually accompany irregular ovulation.

During a period, a woman usually sheds between two and four tablespoons of blood, some women considerably more. This typically occurs over four to six days, although anything from two to eight days is normal. The cramp-like discomfort or pain is usually confined to the first day, but commonly continues for two, three or sometimes more days.

As most women know only too well, even normal healthy periods can cause quite a lot of misery. The most common complaints are PMS (premenstrual syndrome), severe period pains, heavy or prolonged periods, or irregular periods.

PMS – premenstrual syndrome

Over 150 different symptoms have been blamed on the hormonal changes in the few days before each period. The commonest are tension, irritability, depression (sometimes severe enough to be suicidal), fatigue, headaches, poor concentration, clumsiness, feeling bloated, swelling of the face, hands, feet, breasts and abdomen, various aches and pains, and disturbances of sleep. One or more of these could constitute PMS providing that the symptoms disappear within a day or two of starting a period.

About one woman in three (of reproductive age) has some form of premenstrual disturbance or discomfort – but only about one in twenty seeks treatment for it, usually when they are in their thirties or early forties.

PMS is thought to be caused by fluid and salt retention triggered by the hormonal changes at that time in the menstrual cycle (high oestrogen and low progesterone levels).

There are various ways in which you can help to minimise the disturbance PMS can bring.

- **Explain the problem to your family and workmates – so that they can understand and be supportive**
- **Rearrange important or demanding dates to avoid your worst days**
- **Learn a few simple relaxation techniques such as deep breathing (see pp. 67–8)**
- **Try cutting down on salt and salty foods**
- **Try a mild diuretic (to increase fluid loss). Ask your pharmacist.**
- **Consider going on the Pill**
- **Try vitamin B6 (pyridoxine) and/or evening primrose oil**
- **If all else fails, see your doctor – various hormonal treatments can usually help.**

Period pains

Every woman of reproductive age expects some discomfort on the first day of her period, but about one woman in every three has quite severe pain, perhaps lasting into the second or third day, or beyond that.

There are two main types of painful periods (dysmenorrhoea). The commonest begins at puberty and goes on until the first pregnancy, usually easing considerably when periods restart after childbirth. It is felt mainly in the lower abdomen, back and thighs – gnawing, dragging, cramps.

The other type occurs in older women and may be caused by various gynaecological disorders such as fibroids (non-cancerous growths in the womb), endometriosis (womb-lining tissue which has spread to other parts of the pelvic cavity), or ovarian cysts. It can also be caused by the coil.

You can help yourself by resting on your side with your legs tucked up and a hot water bottle on your tummy. If ordinary painkillers such as aspirin, paracetamol or ibuprofen don't help, try one of the special formulations (usually containing codeine and/or caffeine) from the chemist.

Many women find that Vitamin B6 and evening primrose oil are helpful with period pains as well as PMS. Rhythmic exercise can help too – especially skipping, bouncing and jogging.

In severe cases in younger women, going on the Pill can bring relief, but the pains usually return when you come off it again. If you're an older woman or your periods are particularly heavy as well as painful, it's best to see your doctor for a check-up and perhaps special hormonal treatment.

Heavy or prolonged periods

Also known as menorrhagia. The amount of menstrual flow depends mainly on how thickly the inner lining of your womb grows each month. This will vary with the duration of your cycle – a longer one usually means a heavier period. Also, the larger your womb, the more tissue to expel and the fuller the flow. A single heavy period after unprotected sex may actually be a miscarriage.

The whole menstrual cycle depends on perfect harmony between your hormone system, your general metabolism, your state of health and your emotions. Quite a balancing act. It's easily knocked out of kilter by such things as crash dieting, illness, worry or a change of routine. Obesity can have an effect too – the excess body fat takes up oestrogen and not enough may be available to allow regular ovulation.

In older women, the approaching menopause can cause heavy periods or 'flooding'. Really heavy periods in younger women may mean a more severe hormone imbalance, such as that caused by polycystic ovaries (i.e. ovaries with many cysts).

You can often help to regulate your periods by maintaining a healthy lifestyle – with a varied, balanced diet (including lots of fresh fruit and vegetables), frequent physical activity, and regular sleep.

For the great majority of younger women who seek medical treatment, the Pill helps greatly by regulating the cycle. Older women may also be helped by hormonal treatment, but it's usually advisable for them to have a D & C (dilatation and curettage – or 'scrape'), to remove any excessive womb lining through the cervix, and perhaps an ultrasound scan to see if there are any large fibroids or other pelvic problems. Women with heavy periods may need extra iron to prevent or correct anaemia.

Irregular periods

This too is a very common problem and doesn't usually indicate any abnormality, just a variation on the regular pattern of ovulation. The main reasons for periods going haywire have been mentioned above, but many women have irregular periods from puberty onwards for no apparent reason. It often takes two or three years for the cycle to settle down to a regular pattern. Exams, emotional upsets, dieting, and heavy physical training can all upset it.

Irregular periods in themselves may not cause too much trouble, but they are often heavy as well. Sometimes they are scanty and very few and far between. Sometimes a period may be missed completely, perhaps causing a bit of a scare. Such irregularities are common in younger women on strict diets, or those who have anorexia. It may also happen for several months after coming off the Pill or after childbirth. In older women, the periods usually become irregular and less frequent, often with flooding, in the years approaching the menopause. Occasionally, irregular periods may be caused by abnormal hormonal disturbances because of polycystic ovaries.

In younger women, apart from maintaining a healthy lifestyle (especially healthy eating with plenty of fresh fruit and vegetables), going on the Pill will regulate the cycle. Older women may need a check-up and D & C as for heavy periods.

HEALTH IN PREGNANCY

If you're trying for a baby, it's important to get yourself into as healthy a state of mind and body as you can. For one thing, you're more likely to conceive successfully if you're in peak health. And secondly, the first few days of an embryo's existence are crucial for the future baby's health, which very much depends on the nutritional and chemical environment in which the embryo finds itself.

A healthy conception

So, for your baby's sake as well as your own, you need to follow all the advice given earlier in this book about healthy eating, exercise, smoking, drinking and drugs *whilst you're still trying to conceive*. This is far better than waiting until you know you're pregnant. It's particularly beneficial to come off any strict slimming diet you may be on, and to stop or cut right down on smoking and alcoholic drinks.

There is one particular vitamin you should have more of whilst you're trying to get pregnant. This is folic acid, which helps prevent spina bifida and other serious problems in the developing embryo. You should take folic acid tablets (in a dose of 400 microgrammes daily) before you conceive and until you are twelve weeks pregnant, and then stop.

Nutrition in pregnancy

Contrary to popular belief, you don't have to 'eat for two' when you're pregnant. During the first three months, you'll need only an extra 150 calories a day, rising to an extra 350 calories a day during the last six months.

Even so, you will find that your appetite is increased, and it's important to eat the right things – the healthy balance of foods outlined in Chapter 1 – rather than scoffing masses of fried food, biscuits, cakes and chocolates. This is not dieting – it's sensible eating. You must expect to gain quite a bit of weight during pregnancy – on average about two stone (13kg) – but this is normal and natural and important for your health as well as your baby's. If you're concerned about putting on much more than that, talk to your midwife or GP. But remember that too little weight gain in pregnancy is usually more of a worry than too much.

What you should eat during pregnancy
- **Plenty of fruit and vegetables.**
  These help to provide the vitamins and minerals you and your baby need, as well as fibre, which helps digestion and prevents constipation. Wash them thoroughly and eat them lightly cooked or raw to get the most out of them. Frozen and tinned fruit and vegetables are good too.

- More starchy foods like bread, potatoes, rice, pasta and breakfast cereals. These help to satisfy your hunger without containing too many calories. They are also an important source of vitamins and fibre.
- Lean meat, fish, eggs, cheese, beans and lentils. All good sources of nutrients. Eat some every day.
- Dairy products like milk, cheese and yoghurt. Important because they contain calcium and other nutrients needed for your baby's development.
- Cut down on sugar and sugary things, and also fat, fried foods and other fatty things. Look for low-fat versions of dairy products, for example semi-skimmed or skimmed milk, low-fat yoghurt and half-fat hard cheese. Go easy on salt too.

Vitamins and minerals

- Green leafy vegetables, lean red meat, dried fruits and nuts contain *iron*. If you're short of iron you're likely to get very tired and may suffer from anaemia.
- Citrus fruit, tomatoes, broccoli, blackcurrants and potatoes are good sources of Vitamin C which you need to help you to absorb iron.
- Dairy products, fish with edible bones like sardines, bread, nuts and green vegetables are rich in calcium – vital for making bones and teeth.
- Margarines or oily fish (like tinned sardines) contain Vitamin D to help you absorb *calcium*. But the best source of Vitamin D is sunlight, so try to get out for a while every day.
- Before you get pregnant, and for the first twelve weeks of pregnancy, you need extra *folic acid*. This helps to prevent your baby having spina bifida and other serious problems. You can get folic acid from green leafy vegetables, and from breakfast cereals and breads which have had folic acid added to them. Check the labels.

Take care with some foods

Besides eating a wide variety of foods, there are certain precautions you will need to take in order to safeguard your baby's well-being as well as your own:

- Make sure eggs are thoroughly cooked until the whites and yolks are solid, to prevent the risk of salmonella food poisoning.

- Avoid eating all types of pâté and ripened soft cheese, like brie and camembert, as well as goat and sheep milk cheese and blue-veined cheese, because of the risk of listeria infection.
- Drink only pasteurised or UHT milk which have had the harmful germs destroyed. If only green-top (raw) milk is available, boil it before you drink.
- Don't eat liver or liver products – like liver pâté or liver sausage – as they contain a lot of Vitamin A. Too much Vitamin A could harm your baby.
- Have caffeine-containing drinks in moderation – like coffee, tea and colas. There may be a slight risk that too much caffeine could affect your baby's birthweight. Switch to decaffeinated coffee, fruit juice or mineral water.

Extra vitamins?

If you follow the sensible eating advice here, you shouldn't need any vitamin supplements apart from folic acid. Don't take any other extra vitamins or minerals without your doctor's advice. Beware of Vitamin A supplements – too much Vitamin A could harm your baby.

Smoking and pregnancy

When you smoke, carbon monoxide and nicotine passes into your lungs and bloodstream, and through the placenta into your baby. This means that your baby gets less oxygen and can't grow as well as it should. There are other effects too.

But if you stop smoking:

- you're more likely to have a healthier pregnancy, and a healthier baby
- you'll cope better with the birth
- your baby will cope better with any birth complication
- your baby is less likely to be born too early and have to face the breathing, feeding and other health problems that premature birth so often leads to
- your baby is less likely to be born underweight. Low birthweight babies are more prone to infections and have trouble keeping warm.

The sooner you stop, the better. So go for it and follow the guidelines in Chapter 4. If anyone else at home smokes, get them to join you – even their smoke can affect you and the baby.

Alcohol

There's no evidence that very light or occasional drinking during pregnancy is likely to harm your baby. But research shows that heavy or frequent drinking certainly can cause your baby all sorts of serious problems.

To be on the safe side, stop altogether or stick to no more than one 'unit of alcohol' (see p. 80) once or twice a *week*. Instead, there are plenty of non-alcoholic or low-alcohol drinks to enjoy. If you have difficulty cutting down, follow the advice in Chapter 4.

Pills, medicines and other drugs

Many medications are potentially harmful for the baby in the womb. The sensible course of action is to:

- **assume all medications are dangerous until a doctor or pharmacist can tell you they are safe in pregnancy**
- **make sure your doctor or dentist knows you're pregnant before they prescribe you anything or give you X-rays or treatment. The same applies if you have to go to hospital for any reason**
- **talk to your doctor at the first possible moment if you take regular medication.**

Illegal street drugs can also be very harmful for your baby, especially cocaine or crack which can cause a sudden drop in oxygen to the placenta. If you need advice, see your doctor or call a drugs helpline.

Other hazards

Animals: Cat faeces may contain an organism which causes toxoplasmosis, a disease which, though mild in adults, can damage the unborn baby. While you're pregnant, avoid emptying cat litter trays. Don't touch sick cats or those with kittens (including the kittens). Wear gloves when gardening because of possible contact with cat faeces. Always wash your hands thoroughly after handling any cat.

Lambs and sheep can be the source of an organism which may cause mis-carriage. Avoid lambing or milking ewes and all contact with newborn lambs.

Work: If you work with chemicals, solvents, lead, X-rays, or you're in a job with a lot of lifting, you may be risking your health and that of your unborn baby. It's best to discuss any worries you may have about work hazards with your doctor, or the occupational health staff, union reps or personnel department.

Some women are concerned about earlier reports of the possible effects of VDUs (visual display units or computer screens) on their pregnancy. However, the latest research shows no evidence of any risk.

Physical Activity and Pregnancy

The more active and fit you are, the easier it will be to cope comfortably with your changing size and shape during pregnancy – and to bounce back afterwards.

Keep up your normal daily physical activity or exercise – whether it be sport, dancing, just walking to the shops and back, or whatever you're used to – even do a little more than you're used to, as long as you feel comfortable. Never exhaust yourself and, if necessary, slow down as pregnancy progresses, or if your midwife or doctor advises you to. Stick to the basic principles for healthy physical activity outlined in Chapter 2.

In later pregnancy, there are a few special exercises that are worth fitting into your daily routine:

- **Foot exercises to improve your circulation and help prevent leg cramps and swollen ankles. With your legs straight, bend and stretch your feet vigorously up and down fifty times. Rotate your feet ten times in one direction, ten times in the other.**
- **Pelvic rocking to strengthen abdominal muscles and ease backache. Kneel on all fours, arch your back, pull in your tummy and look at your knees. Now slowly relax your back and raise your head. Repeat ten times.**
- **Pelvic floor exercises to strengthen the muscles of the pelvic floor, which are greatly stretched and strained during late pregnancy and childbirth. This is the usual cause of 'stress incontinence', the leaky bladder so many women get after they've had a baby. You can do the exercises anywhere, surreptitiously. Simply tighten your back passage as if preventing a bowel movement and at the same time draw in your vagina and urethra. Hold the muscles clenched like this for ten seconds and relax. Repeat ten times in quick succession, and do this five or ten sessions a day.**

Sex in pregnancy

There's no reason why you shouldn't carry on having sex all the way through your pregnancy if you want to. It doesn't harm the baby – the cervix seals off the womb completely.

The main exception to this is if you've had a miscarriage, in which case it's probably best to avoid intercourse in the first four months.

In later pregnancy, if you have an orgasm it may set off contractions – but this is perfectly normal and doesn't mean you're about to give birth. If it feels uncomfortable just lie quietly for a few minutes until the contractions subside.

At the very end of pregnancy, you should definitely not have intercourse once the waters have broken.

After the birth

Try to take things easy for a while, and get your partner, family and friends to help you manage at home. Try to have a sleep or proper rest at least once a day.

Continue with the post-natal exercises you were shown in hospital. Also, do your pelvic floor exercises, as described above.

You could also do the following tummy tightening exercise three or four times a day. And go for walks with your baby – it'll make you both feel good.

Tummy tightener
- Lie on your back with your knees bent
- Curl your head and shoulders from the floor and reach towards your feet with both hands
- Hold for a few seconds and then relax
- Repeat ten times, increasing to twenty.

A HEALTHY MENOPAUSE

Women vary greatly in their experience of the menopause – physically and emotionally.

For four out of five, it's something which bothers them little or not at all – they sail through it, hardly noticing what's happening to them.

But for the rest, it can mean any of a whole catalogue of miseries.

What sets it off?

The ovaries begin to 'wind down' from the late thirties onwards – although this is barely noticeable at first. Between the ages of about forty-five and fifty-five, dwindling levels of female hormones begin to cause some iregularity of ovulation and periods – a process accelerated by cigarette smoking. Usually the periods become less frequent and lighter, although sometimes bouts of heavier bleeding can occur ('flooding'). However, frequent heavy periods, clots, or bleeding between periods are not normal, and any woman with these should see her doctor for a check-up.

Because of 'missed' periods, many women find themselves wondering if they may be pregnant. In fact, as ovulation becomes increasingly sporadic, their ability to conceive fades rapidly.

After an average of five or six years, the periods stop altogether – although they may drag on for up to twice that length of time, or, in some cases, cease in as little as six months flat. All the while, the levels of oestrogen and progesterone fall steadily.

What are the main problems?

The most common is hot flushes – an unpleasant feeling of heat in the chest, sweeping up over the face and arms. They can be mild or severe, occasional or frequent, and can happen day or night (when they may be accompanied by 'drenches' or night sweats). They're often triggered by hot drinks and spicy food, alcohol, or embarrassment. Sometimes they're linked to a panic attack. Most women have flushes for about a year, then they begin to ease off.

Another common problem is vaginal dryness – a distressing symptom which many women interpret as the end of their sex life, because penetration becomes difficult and painful. The dryness is owing to a lack of normal vaginal secretions and may be accompanied by attacks of thrush (candida, a fungal irritation), painful urination and cystitis, or itching of the vulva.

Understandably, many women feel tense and irritable during their menopause, others are weepy and depressed. Phobias are common, particularly agoraphobia (fear of going out, especially to crowded places). So too are panic attacks. All these changes are linked to the dwindling hormone levels.

Other problems include headaches, dizziness, insomnia, fatigue, lack of energy, abdominal distension, irritable bowels, palpitations and breathlessness. As time goes by, the lack of oestrogen leads to a thinning and drying of the skin and hair, weakening of the pelvic floor muscles (which may cause a prolapse), and an increase in cholesterol which puts up the risk of heart disease and osteoporosis.

Osteoporosis

Oestrogen and other hormones play an important part in the balance of calcium in your bones. As oestrogen levels subside with the menopause and beyond in later life, the bones lose calcium and become thinner and weaker. This makes them very vulnerable to fractures after knocks or falls.

Although osteoporosis occurs in older men too, it happens much sooner and more rapidly in women and is about four times as common. The earlier your menopause, the more likely osteoporosis is.

Contraception and the menopause

The usual advice is that, for women under fifty, you should continue contraception for a year after your last period – and, for women over fifty, for six months.

Self-help

- **Hot flushes** – Try to avoid the trigger situations – not always easy, since even a cup of tea can bring one on. But you can avoid spicy food, cut down on alcohol, wear light clothing and keep as cool as possible.

- **Vaginal dryness** – Use a lubricant jelly from the chemist (but warm it first!). Thrush should be treated with antifungal cream or suppositories also obtainable without prescription from chemists, but see your doctor if you're not sure it's thrush.

- **Emotional problems** – Try to understand that this is a temporary phase in your life, and that there is light at the end of the tunnel. Life can be just as good beyond the menopause. Think positive, be more active. Your partner, family and friends can help by being sympathetic and understanding. Follow the relaxation advice in Chapter 4.

- **Osteoporosis** – Take up regular physical exercise, preferably before your menopause, but as soon as you can. Choose activities which use your legs and bear your weight – like walking, dancing, tennis – to strengthen the bones in your back, hips, knees and feet. Follow the advice in Chapter 3. Make sure you have enough calcium – there's plenty in low fat dairy products.

The great majority of women going through the menopause don't need hormone replacement therapy. It is a myth to think of it as an elixir of youth. Nevertheless, in selected cases with particular menopausal problems, HRT can, without doubt, make a big difference.

Severe debilitating hot flushes or night sweats, distressing vaginal changes, high cholesterol, osteoporosis and some of the emotional problems can be relieved or reduced by monthly courses of oestrogen and progestogen (an artificial progesterone). This treatment closely mimics a woman's natural hormonal cycle, and on HRT she will continue to have monthly 'periods' (although she will no longer be ovulating). HRT can be taken as pills, skin patches, implanted pellets or, for vaginal changes, as a vaginal cream.

Apart from continuing periods, the snags with HRT are that it can cause nausea and breast tenderness, and there may be an increased risk of thrombosis.

The combined form of HRT does not increase the risk of uterine (womb) cancer but, after several years, the risk of breast cancer may be higher. For these reasons, HRT can only be given on prescription, and needs careful follow-up checks. Doctors vary greatly in their recommendations for HRT. Some advocate just six to twelve months' treatment, others up to ten years or so.

BREAST AWARENESS

Every woman knows it's important for her to be aware of any changes in her breasts, and to see her doctor if she notices anything unusual. But what does unusual mean? Which changes are normal and which need a check-up? And what does breast screening involve?

The trouble with breasts is that they are such variable organs – not so much in the way they differ in size and shape from woman to woman (although that's certainly true enough), but in the way they change throughout the menstrual cycle. This fluctuation not only causes discomfort for many women, but also makes it more difficult to detect abnormal changes.

Normal monthly changes

In the second half of the cycle the breasts slowly become a little larger, partly due to engorgement of the breast glands and ducts, and partly to fluid retention in the connective tissue surrounding them. Many women feel a fullness and dragging heaviness in their breasts as their period approaches, perhaps even discomfort or pain. At the same time the breasts have a lumpy or gritty feel to them. Then, with the onset of menstruation, the engorgement and lumpiness subside, and the breasts return to their comfortable state again.

Breast tenderness

About one woman in three experiences this monthly discomfort, and for many it's severe enough for them to seek help from their doctor. Some women have the problem for three of the four weeks of their menstrual cycle. No position is comfortable, and many activities, such as walking (especially up and down stairs) and lovemaking, are so painful that they are avoided as much as possible. The problem not only interferes with work and leisure, but also puts considerable strain on sexual relations.

Other causes of pain in the breast area include a pulled or bruised chest muscle, or, in older women, wear and tear of the spine, causing pressure on a nerve supplying the breast area. Breast cancer can sometimes reveal itself as a localised tenderness, but this is relatively unusual.

What can you do about tender breasts? Try these simple self-help measures:

- **Wear a good supporting bra – even at night if it helps.**
- **Take a simple painkiller like soluble aspirin, paracetamol or ibuprofen.**
- **Try Vitamin B6 (pyridoxine) in the week or so before each period.**
- **Evening primrose oil capsules may help too.**
- **You may find that cutting down on tea and coffee is beneficial.**
- **If these simple steps don't help, or the pain is on one side only, see your doctor.**

Breast lumps

Generalised lumpiness throughout the breast tissue is normal in the second half of the menstrual cycle, particularly in smaller, less fatty breasts. But if you think you can feel a single lump, whether tender or not, you should get it properly checked without delay.

Far and away the most likely cause of a lump is a cyst in a blocked gland or duct owing to benign breast disease, the name given to monthly lumpiness which is severe enough not to subside completely with each period.

Another less common cause is the more mobile type of lump known as a fibroadenoma or 'breast mouse', so called because it is mobile enough to manoeuvre around the breast tissue.

The third, and least likely cause of a lump is breast cancer, which is usually not tender and is fixed rather then mobile.

If your doctor agrees that there's a lump that needs a proper check-up to ensure that it isn't cancer, you'll be referred to the breast specialist at your local hospital.

Breast screening

'Screening' is the term used for checking large numbers of people for evidence of a disease before any symptoms have appeared. The idea is to detect the disease, or some condition that precedes it, as early as possible, long before it becomes noticeable. This way, there's a much better chance of preventing or curing it.

Screening for breast cancer can save your life. It's the most common cancer in women, and the risk increases as you get older, especially over the age of fifty. In Britain, the NHS offers a three-yearly breast screening service to women aged between fifty and sixty-four. An invitation is sent to all women in this age-group who are registered with a GP, and the service is free. For women of sixty-five or over, the service is available on request.

The screening test is a mammogram – a very low-dose X-ray of the breasts. Each breast is flattened gently against a special plate and the X-ray taken. Although this may be slightly uncomfortable, it's all over in seconds. If you're in the age bracket for breast screening, and you receive an invitation, make sure you accept it and go for screening. It's well worth doing for your peace of mind.

How to examine your breasts

It's a good idea to get into the habit of examining your breasts once a month, in the fortnight after your period if you have periods.

- **Undressed to the waist, sit or stand in front of a mirror, arms by your sides. Look for any change in appearance – any puckering or dimpling of the skin, any change in the outline, any discharge or bleeding from the nipple.**
- **Now raise your arms above your head. Does a pucker or dimple appear?**
- **Put your hands on your hips and push. Again, any pucker or dimple?**
- **Now, lie down on the bed with a folded towel under one shoulder and that arm above your head to stretch your breast. With the *flat* of the other hand (not the fingertips), gently feel each imaginary quarter of the breast, from the edge of the breast to the nipple. Also feel the armpit.**
- **Repeat with the other breast.**

> **Consult your doctor if you notice:**
> - any unusual puckering or dimpling.
> - any change in outline or shape.
> - any indrawing or distortion of the nipple.
> - any discharge or bleeding from the nipple.
> - any rash around the nipple.
> - any unusually prominent veins.
> - any lump or unusual tenderness.
> - anything else that bothers you.

VAGINAL HEALTH

Natural cleansing

Many women are unnecessarily anxious about the health and hygiene of their vagina, thinking they have to douche it frequently to keep it clean and odour-free.

In fact, the vagina is very good at looking after itself. The normal vaginal secretion is the most natural and effective cleansing agent, having an anti-microbial action and the correct slightly acid pH to help control bacteria and fungi. Douching is not a good idea because it removes this natural defence.

Normal secretion

The composition of your vaginal secretion is influenced by your hormonal balance and will vary greatly according to your time of month, whether you're on the Pill, whether you're pregnant, or whether you've been through the menopause.

In most women, the secretion increases at mid-cycle (between periods) around the time of ovulation. This type of excess secretion is whitish (or very pale yellow) and may be enough to stain underwear. It may have a slight natural aroma. But providing it's not irritating, and causes no soreness, it's quite normal.

Vaginal discharge

Any change in the normal vaginal secretion can be very worrying for a woman. Apart from the discomfort or embarrassment, there's always the fear that it might be because of a sexually transmitted infection, perhaps with a risk of damage to the tubes, and hence infertility. Small wonder then that vaginal discharge prompts more visits to the doctor than almost any other personal health problem.

If you develop a discharge that is unusual for you – perhaps because there's much more of it, or it smells different, or especially if it's making you itchy or sore – then that isn't normal and may mean you need treatment.

What are the causes?

By far the most common cause is candida or thrush, a yeast-like fungus often present in normal vaginal secretions. Most of the time it causes no trouble – but, for various reasons, it can multiply profusely, which irritates the vagina both inside and out, making it red and sore. The discharge may only be slight, with creamy white specks or 'curds', but the itching can be unbearable.

Thrush is triggered if the normal acidity of the vagina is reduced, as happens during and after each period or during pregnancy. It can also occur if the normal friendly acid-making bacteria in the vagina are destroyed by a course of antibiotics, perhaps for a chest infection. Poorly controlled diabetes encourages thrush by increasing the sugar content of the vagina.

Thrush may also be spread from the bowel, through poor hygiene, and also from a sexual partner.

What about other infections?

The two most likely to cause vaginal discharge are trichomonas vaginalis (TV) and bacterial vaginosis (BV).

TV is a micro-organism, transmitted by sexual contact, which can cause a copious watery greenish discharge, often flaring up quite suddenly, and perhaps accompanied by intense itching. The male partner, by contrast, usually has no symptoms at all.

The discharge caused by BV, which may or may not be sexually transmitted, is greyish in colour with a strong fishy smell. Again there's usually discomfort or itching.

Fortunately, none of the infections mentioned so far is likely to do any lasting harm.

Which infections are more worrying?

Two sexually transmsitted infections, chlamydia and gonorrhoea, may damage the tubes and cause infertility – but they don't usually cause a discharge. Indeed they're unlikely to cause any symptoms in women until it's too late. They're both caught from men who suffer discomfort on passing water and may have a slight discharge from the penis (NSU – non-specific urethritis). Needless to say, it's very important for men with these symptoms to avoid intercourse and to tell their partners to have a check-up.

What's the treatment?

If you have a discharge that's unusual for you, see your doctor or book yourself an appointment at the hospital genito-urinary clinic (no doctor's letter necessary).

Thrush, TV or BV can all be controlled with special medication, given either as pessaries (vaginal tablets) or cream. Chlamydia or gonorrhoea can also be cleared up with a course of antibiotics. Partners should be treated as well.

Flare-ups of thrush can often be prevented by wearing light loose underwear, and avoiding bath salts and strong soap.

CYSTITIS

The chances are you'll suffer from cystitis at some time in your life. Although it's often just a minor discomfort for a day or two, for many women it spells real misery, and has a nasty habit of coming back again and again.

Cystitis is an inflamed bladder – or more accurately, the lining of the bladder. The first symptom is a niggling need to pass water – even though you may have only just done so. You sit there, trying to empty your bladder completely – but nothing happens because there's no more urine left in it. It just *feels* as if there is. A while later, when you do manage to pass a little, it stings your urinary outlet.

The next symptom is a nasty dragging pain in the depths of your lower abdomen or perhaps your lower back. After a day or two, your urine may look cloudy or smoky, or you may see blood in it, and you may feel shivery and feverish.

What causes cystitis?

It's usually caused by an infection – bacteria spreading up the lining of the urinary outlet tube and into the bladder. Normally the waterworks are germ-free, and so too is the urine itself. But the nooks, crannies and secretions of the outer vagina are the perfect breeding ground for bacteria, and it's all too easy for a few to get into the urinary outlet and travel the inch or so into the bladder. Once there, the infection makes the bladder-lining sore and sensitive – hence the constant desire to pass water.

Sexual intercourse, tampon removal, and poor hygiene may all be causes of cystitis – but most cases happen for no obvious reason. Some types aren't caused by infection at all. So-called 'honeymoon cystitis', for example, is caused by friction from over-enthusiastic lovemaking; 'chemical cystitis' from irritant substances in bath gels, perfumed soaps and deodorants.

What can be done about it?

To deal with an attack, day or night, drink a pint of water, milk or weak tea as soon as you feel the first tingle of discomfort. If germs are to blame, this will help to flush them out before they can get a real grip.

If you start to feel the awful ache deep in your pelvis, take two soluble aspirin, paracetamol or ibuprofen tablets, and put a hot-water bottle on your belly, back or between your legs – wherever you find it helps. All three places if you've got enough hot-water bottles!

If you've got some baking powder (sodium bicarbonate) handy, put a teaspoonful in a pint of water or fruit squash, and drink it. Repeat this every hour for three hours. The purpose of the bicarbonate is to neutralise the acidity of your urine, which soothes the stinging and discourages the acid-loving bacteria. Most women find this simple routine relieves their cystitis within three or four hours. However, if you've been diagnosed as having high blood pressure, you should avoid sodium – so leave out the bicarbonate and just drink plain fluid.

What can the doctor do?

If your cystitis has dragged on for more than a day or two, if you're getting repeated attacks, if your urine is cloudy or smoky, if you're feeling feverish, or if you're pregnant – see your doctor. It's important not to let the cystitis get too established because there's a risk of infection spreading up to the kidneys. If a young girl gets cystitis, the risk of kidney infection is much higher and she should be taken to the doctor straight away.

The medical treatment for cystitis is a course of antibiotics. It's important to complete the course even after the symptoms have subsided, to make sure all the bacteria have been killed.

To prevent further attacks, drink plenty of water and soft drinks, and be even more scrupulous about personal hygiene. If you think it may be an allergy, try unperfumed soap and avoid bath oils and gels.

Self-help

1. At the first sign of an attack, drink a pint of water or squash.

2. Repeat this every hour for three or four hours.

3. If possible, add a teaspoonful of sodium bicarbonate to each pint (unless you have high blood pressure).

4. Put a hot-water bottle on your tummy, back or between your legs to ease the ache. Take simple painkillers if necessary.

5. See your doctor if the attack persists for more than a day or two, or you feel feverish.

6. Young girls should be taken to the doctor straight away.

7. If prescribed antibiotics, make sure you complete the full course.

A HEALTHY CERVIX

Various conditions can affect the cervix, the small, dome-like neck of the womb, projecting into the ceiling of the vagina. Far and away the most common are thrush (candida), genital warts, herpes and a cervical erosion. Cervical cancer is relatively unusual, even in older women.

Each of these conditions may or may not cause any symptoms, and are often first diagnosed at a routine cervical smear examination. However, if you experience sharp discomfort or pain on intercourse, felt deep in your pelvis, or notice bleeding after sex, between periods or after the menopause, then you should see your doctor for a check-up without delay.

Cervical screening

This is a simple test – the cervical 'smear' test – which can not only detect cancer before it causes any symptoms, but can also detect cells which might become cancer at some time in the future. Thanks to the cervical smear test and national screening programme, the number of women dying from cervical cancer in Britain is steadily going down.

The usual type of cervical cancer only occurs in women who have had sexual intercourse at some time in their lives, and is almost certainly linked to some sexually transmitted organism. The likeliest culprit is the genital wart virus, which is very widespread among sexually active adults – although they usually carry it without suffering any genital warts. There are over forty strains of this virus, but only a few seem to be associated with an increased risk of cervical cancer.

To complicate matters further, a woman's risk depends on her resistance to the cancer-inducing effect of the virus – some women are more susceptible than others. Smoking, for instance, reduces the body's resistance, increasing the risk of cervical cancer.

In general, the earlier a woman becomes sexually active, and the more partners she has, the more at risk she is. This risk increases steadily as she gets older, even though she may subsequently have one faithful partner, or her sex life may have long since come to an end.

Can it be prevented?

Fortunately, yes. First, by using a condom, which helps to protect against the wart virus. And secondly, by having regular smear tests to detect changes that occur before cancer develops.

These abnormal changes in the cells of the cervix are called dysplasia, and there are very effective treatments to remove a patch of dysplasia long before it has the chance to turn into cancer.

In Britain, all women aged twenty to sixty-four registered with a GP are automatically invited to have a regular smear test – and it may also be offered at family planning or postnatal clinics. Needless to say, the test is very worthwhile. It simply involves a brief 'internal' examination, and a gentle wipe of the cervix with a wooden or plastic spatula to pick up some mucus.

What is a 'positive' smear?

In the great majority of cases it does not mean you've got cancer. If confirmed with a repeat smear, it means that some cells are dysplastic – over a period of years they could eventually become malignant, though not necessarily.

What's the treatment?

Women with very mild changes may simply be asked to have a repeat smear every six months to keep an eye on things. With less mild changes, the cervix usually needs inspecting closely through a colposcope (special binoculars) and a pinhead-sized sample taken.

If a patch of dysplasia is confirmed, it can be destroyed either by a freeze probe, a heat probe, or a laser, under local anaesthetic.

A small proportion of women have severe dysplasia, and need a wedge of cervix removed under general anaesthetic. Fortunately this heals well and usually causes no problems with conception or pregnancy.

The few women who are found to have actual invasive cancer will need a special hysterectomy and radiotherapy or chemotherapy to destroy any lingering cancer cells.

TRAVEL WELL

So, it's all fixed. You've got your holiday all booked up, or business trip arranged, and you'll soon be up-up-and-away to some far-flung exotic paradise, lying on a sun-drenched beach, dipping in the warm blue sea, dawdling through the market, or tasting the delights of the local cuisine.

But, caution. Many is the holiday or business trip marred by the nausea of motion sickness, a gut-squirming tummy upset, searing sunburn, or some utterly prostrating tropical fever that lingers for weeks after you get back. If you get back!

As everyone knows, travel can damage your health – or at least give it a nasty jolt. But with a bit of care and forethought – before you go, in transit, and whilst you're there – there's every chance you'll be able to avoid the main pitfalls and have a happy, healthy time away.

BEFORE YOU GO

The golden rule is to plan as far ahead of your trip as you can, particularly if you're going anywhere tropical or subtropical. Just because the brochure boasts luxury hotels, first class restaurants, air-conditioned touring facilities and experienced guides, doesn't mean you can't be bitten by a malaria-carrying mosquito, pick up hepatitis in the market or succumb to dysentery from the drinking water.

Vaccinations

For travel to anywhere outside Europe, the US, Canada, Australia or New Zealand, you'll almost certainly need various vaccinations, some of which may be essential to enter particular countries with their own special vaccination requirements.

It can take up to six weeks to complete the courses of some types of vaccination. So, as soon as you know which countries you'll be visiting or travelling through, ask your travel agent, airline or the embassy concerned for details of which vaccinations you'll be needing, either because they're essential or recommended. At the same time, ask about malaria and other health risks. It's

	Disease risk areas	*How caught*
AIDS	World-wide	From having sex with an infected person; from injections with infected blood or needles.
Cholera	Africa, Asia, Middle East, especially in conditions of poor hygiene and sanitation.	From contaminated food or water.
Viral Hepatitis A	Most parts of the world but especially in conditions of poor hygiene and sanitation.	From contaminated food or water.
Viral Hepatitis B	World-wide.	By intimate contact with an infected person; from injections with infected blood or needles (as AIDS).
Malaria	Africa, Asia, Central and South America.	Bite from infected mosquito.
Poliomyelitis	Everywhere except Australia, New Zealand, Europe and North America.	Direct contact with an infected person; rarely by contaminated water or food.
Rabies	Many parts of the world.	Bite or scratch from an infected animal.
Tetanus	World-wide but particularly dangerous in places where medical facilities are not readily available.	Any skin-penetrating wound, especially if soiled.
Tuberculosis	Asia, Africa, Central and South America.	Airborne from infectious person.
Typhoid	Everywhere except Australia, New Zealand, Europe, North America, in conditions of poor hygiene and sanitation.	Contaminated food, water or milk.
Yellow Fever	Africa and South America.	Bite from infected mosquito.

Smallpox has been eradicated worldwide and there is NO requirement for the vaccination of travellers.

Vaccination	Vaccination certificate needed	Other precautions
None available.	No, but some countries have introduced HIV antibody testing for some visitors (or require an HIV antibody test certificate for some visitors. See note below.)	Using a condom (rubber or sheath) during sex gives some protection. Take a travel kit for use in medical emergencies.
Usually 2 injections by your doctor.	Some countries may require evidence of vaccination. Certificate valid for 6 months.	Vaccination gives modest protection only, so take scrupulous care over food and drink.
Immunoglobulin if not already immune.	No.	Take scrupulous care over food and drink.
Your doctor will advise on the need for vaccination.	No.	Avoid casual unprotected sexual or other intimate contact.
None, but anti-malarial tablets are available.	No.	Insect repellants, burning coils, pellets, mosquito nets.
Drops by mouth in 3 doses (spacing depends upon age). Reinforcing dose advised after 10 years.	No.	Take scrupulous care over food and drink.
Vaccination may be advised **after** a bite. Get advice from a doctor immediately.	No.	
Vaccination is safe, effective and gives long-lasting protection.	No.	Wash the wound thoroughly and consult a doctor without delay.
Skin test and injection at least 2 months before travel.	No.	Seek medical advice for chest pain, persistent cough or sputum, especially if bloodstained.
2 injections from your doctor, 4-6 weeks apart. Revaccination by 1 injection usually after 3 years.	No.	Take scrupulous care over food and drink.
1 injection at a yellow fever vaccination centre at least 10 days before you go abroad.	Yes. Certificate valid for 10 years.	Avoid mosquito bites, as for malaria.

Note: If in doubt about HIV antibody test certificate requirements, check the current position with the Embassy or High Commission in London of the country concerned.

(Based on Department of Health recommendations)　　**137**

important to mention if you're pregnant, or taking a baby with you, or if you're on immunosuppressive medication such as steroids.

See your doctor at least two months before departure to arrange the jabs and, if your children are going to be travelling with you, they'll need jabs too.

Malaria

In many parts of Africa, Asia, Central and South America, all it takes is a single bite from an infected mosquito to give you malaria, a serious and sometimes fatal disease.

If necessary, ask your doctor about obtaining malaria tablets. You'll need to start these one week before you travel to a malarious area, the whole time you're there, and for one month after returning (children too).

Medical and dental treatment

Proper medical insurance is essential for all travellers abroad, including children. Reciprocal health care arrangements are available to European residents travelling in other parts of Europe. And similar schemes apply in some other countries. But, these schemes only cover emergency treatment, not ongoing complications. So insurance is crucial, otherwise you could be faced with massive bills for prolonged hospitalisation or the cost of getting you back home. Ask your travel agent, airline or the relevant embassy about this.

Your regular medication

If you're on the Pill or regular medication for some long-term condition, ask your doctor about supplies of this for your trip. You may also need a doctor's letter to get them through Customs. If you've got any doubts about your teeth, have a check-up before you leave. Treatment can be hellishly expensive abroad.

Traveller's first aid kit

It all depends where you're going, and what you're going to do when you get there – but here are a few basic items that may be worth their weight in gold.

- Travel sickness pills – the newer types don't cause drowsiness.
- Sunscreen lotion – SPF 15 at least.
- Tablets or capsules for diarrhoea – don't skimp on these.
- Adhesive dressings – mixed shapes and sizes.
- Antiseptic cream.
- Painkillers – paracetamol is a good all-rounder – aspirin helps to lower fevers, but is unsuitable for children under twelve.
- Insect repellent – look for one containing 'deet'.
- Water-sterilisation tablets.
- Rehydration sachets or tablets – especially for babies and small children.
- Tweezers – for splinters, sea-urchin spikes, etc.
- Scissors – for all sorts of things.
- Condoms.

ON THE JOURNEY

OK. You've had an armful of jabs, bought the insurance, and packed a few first-aid essentials. Now, at last, you're on your way. How can you make the going easier?

By air

Ears

Your ears may give you trouble on take-off and landing, especially if you've got a cold or catarrh. Babies and children are even more vulnerable. Try swallowing or yawning to equalise the pressure. Sucking a sweet or chewing gum may help too. Babies can be comforted with a drink. If you're prone to blocked sinuses, take a decongestant before the flight.

Motion sickness

Usually not too much of a problem unless the flight is bumpy. Avoiding alcohol and fatty food may help. But the best answer is to take a travel sickness pill at least half an hour before take-off.

Stiffness and swelling

Long hours in an airline seat may cause your neck, back and joints to stiffen and fluid to collect in your feet. Get up and walk about if you can – but if not, do some simple stretching exercises. Rotate your neck and shoulders, alternately pull in and relax your tummy, and waggle your feet up and down. Loosen your shoelaces or kick off your shoes.

Flying phobia

Try some of the simple relaxation techniques described in Chapter 4, such as deep breathing or progressive relaxation. A drink or two from the bar trolley may help too. Before your next trip, consider a course of hypnotherapy.

By sea

Motion sickness

This is the big worry about a sea crossing. Few people are immune to sea-sickness – and few sea-going craft, even those fitted with stabilisers, are unperturbed by gales and ocean-rollers.

Although there are various tricks to reduce sea-sickness, the best defence is to take an anti-sickness pill about half an hour before leaving harbour. Ask your pharmacist for a type that doesn't cause drowsiness, especially if you've got to drive when you disembark. But don't take them if you're pregnant.

Tips for better sea-legs

- Go up on deck – it helps to see the horizon.
- If you must stay inside – keep to the middle of the boat where there's less pitch and roll.
- Avoid alcohol and fatty foods.
- It may help to lie flat with your eyes shut.
- An anti-sickness pill is the surest precaution.

By vehicle

Motion sickness

Car or coach journeys can be a trial for anyone prone to motion sickness, children in particular. You don't really want to have to dose them up with travel pills for the entire touring holiday.

Discourage children from reading or playing with toys in the back of the car. Try to get them them to look out of the front window if possible, or ahead out of the side. Playing quizzes, spelling games, I-spy, spot-the-tune, or similar distraction, can take their minds off the problem. Nibbling an apple, sipping fruit juice or sucking a sweet may help too. But, if necessary, frequent stops for a run-about may be the best answer.

WHILE YOU'RE THERE

Great! You've arrived in one piece. But, there may still be a few hazards waiting to strike the unwary – the sun, the food and drink, the wild life (in all senses). Here's some advice to minimise the risks.

Safe in the sun?

Why is there always something to spoil life's simple pleasures? Too much food and we get fat. Unsafe sex and we may catch HIV. Basking in the sun and we're prone to sunburn and skin cancer.

These days, we're all very aware of the dangers of too much sun on our skin. Skin cancer is the particular scourge of fairer-skinned people who live in or visit sunny climes. Australia is plagued by it. But even in rain-swept Britain it's the second most common form of cancer, and rapidly increasing. Middle aged and elderly people are most at risk – but the damage is done in youth. Just one bad bout of sunburn in childhood could cause the most dangerous type of skin cancer, melanoma (malignant mole), many years later, although fortunately rarely.

Ultraviolet rays

The culprit is the ultraviolet rays in sunlight. These penetrate to the deeper layers of the skin, denaturing the protein, breaking down the collagen and causing the cells to age rapidly. This makes them more likely to become cancerous.

The fairer or more freckled the skin, and the less easily it tans, the more vulnerable it is. But even people who tan easily increase their risk by spending more time in the sun.

The worst thing is to get sunburnt – especially babies and children. Never let it happen.

Sun sense
- Take care of your skin – it isn't leather – yet!
- Tan slowly, no more than fifteen to twenty minutes a side to start with.
- Avoid the midday sun.
- Use a sunscreen with the right SPF for your skin – at least 15. Reapply it after bathing.
- Never let yourself get sunburnt – if you're pink or tingling, you've overdone it.
- If you don't tan, use a sunblock – or better still, cover up.
- Wear a wide-brimmed hat, loose clothes, and spend more time in the shade.
- Avoid the sun in the middle of the day when the UV rays are at their most damaging.
- Remember, children need extra protection for their more delicate skins.

Molewatch
Watch out for a mole that:

- seems to be getting bigger
- is blotchy or ragged
- weeps or bleeds easily
- is itchy or inflamed
- is larger than the end of a pencil

Any of these could mean a malignant melanoma. If you're not sure about one of your moles, see your doctor without delay.

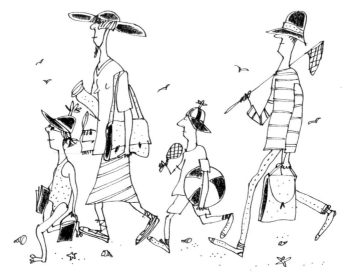

The whole family should wear hats

Heat stroke

All it takes is just a little too long on that Mediterranean beach – despite the lashings of sunscreen – or an hour or two of being jostled in the crowds of a sweltering street market, or playing a few too many games of tennis or volley-ball in the high heat of noon.

Heat stroke has a nasty habit of creeping up on people. The only warning may be a slight feeling of being 'out-of-sorts' with nausea, weariness and a headache. And then, quite suddenly, your skin goes hot and dry and your temperature starts to shoot up through the roof. This is a medical emergency needing urgent treatment – heat stroke can quickly kill. Fortunately, in the great majority of cases, things never get to this dangerous stage. The sufferers are saved by a few simple first aid measures to help them cool down.

Heat stroke is caused by a combination of excessive heat and high humidity – a common situation in many tropical and subtropical areas. In these conditions it's easy to lose several pints of water in a few hours through sweating, and, unless this water is replaced, the sweating mechanism breaks down. If you can no longer sweat, you can't keep cool and your temperature rises out of control.

143

Heat stroke can occur at any age, although older and plumper people are more vulnerable. Holidaymakers are especially at risk because they don't have time to acclimatise properly. Anyone with diarrhoea may succumb to heat exhaustion and heat stroke more easily.

What can be done to help?

1. The crucial thing is to bring the sufferer's temperature down as quickly as possible.

2. It's also important to call for medical attention without delay.

3. Move the sufferer to a cool place in the shade, and remove clothing down to underclothes.

4. Drape a cold, wet sheet or towel over them, or buckets of cold water.

5. Fan the sheet to keep it cool. The more fanning, the better. Make sure you keep the sheet damp.

6. Put some ice cubes in a hanky and place it on the sufferer's forehead.

7. Give sips of iced water to drink.

8. If the sufferer passes out, check they're breathing and turn them face down into the 'recovery' position to keep their airway open until medical help arrives.

Stay cool!

- Wear light, loose clothing made of a natural material such as cotton.
- Spend more time in the shade.
- Put on a wide-brimmed hat in the sun.
- Use a fan if you have one.
- Avoid heavy exertion in the heat of the day.
- Drink plenty of bottled water or soft drinks.
- Put extra salt on your food.

BITES AND STINGS AND OTHER NASTIES

Are you one of those unlucky people who never fail to attract ravaging hordes of midges? Or can't have a picnic without being pulled apart by wood ants? Or live in constant fear of sitting on a bee or swallowing a wasp? Here's a quick guide to help you cope with the little blighters.

1. Insect repellent sprays and creams usually keep midges and mozzies away, but don't deter bees or wasps. Find a brand that works for you, and reapply it every two hours (it's soon diluted by perspiration). Look for one containing 'deet'.

2. Be careful eating fruit and sugary things outdoors – a wasp may have got there first.

3. The best first aid for a wasp- or bee-sting is to hold something cold, like an ice cube, against it. With a bee-sting, remember to flick the sting out first with your nail. Don't try to grab it – you'll squeeze in more poison. Paracetamol (or aspirin for adults) will give long-lasting relief.

4. If you're bitten by ants, ticks, sand-flies or horse-flies, it's best to take an anti-histamine pill.

5. Jellyfish stings can be neutralised with vinegar or lemon juice.

6. Sea urchin spines can be very painful, and fester for weeks. Warn children to keep away from them. If they are pricked, try to remove the broken spines with tweezers, and apply a soothing cream.

7. Watch out for snakes in hot countries. Always carry a torch when walking at night. Don't go barefoot in undergrowth – wear stout shoes and trousers. If someone is bitten, get them to a doctor or hospital as soon as possible.

8. Even in parts of Europe, you could catch rabies if you're bitten, scratched or even licked by an infected dog, cat, fox or other carrier mammal. So, give them a wide berth. If you are attacked, flush the wound immediately with clean water, with or without detergent, and apply neat spirits if available. Get medical attention fast – minutes count.

AVOIDING TUMMY TROUBLES

Even the smartest resorts can play havoc with your innards if you're not careful – especially around the eastern and southern Mediterranean, or anywhere in the tropics. Of course you can't inspect the kitchen of every café or taverna, but here are some simple tips.

1. Avoid drinking tap-water, even in the plushest hotels. Ask for bottled water instead.

2. Peel fruit before you eat it but don't eat fruit which has been peeled for you, especially if it has been sitting around for a while. Wash grapes in drinkable water.

3. Beware 'home-made' ice-cream from street or market vendors. Stick to branded ices.

4. Avoid soft local cheeses, especially if you're pregnant. They may be contaminated with salmonella or listeria.

5. If you're not sure about an eating place, don't accept any meat, poultry, fish or shellfish dish unless it's properly cooked and served piping hot.

6. If you do get the trots, drink plenty of bottled water or fruit juice, adding half a teaspoon of salt per litre to replace losses. Sachets or tablets of rehydration salts are ideal for small children – so make sure you pack a few with you.

JET-LAG

This can be a drag for anyone travelling east–west or west–east between time zones by plane. But it's a special problem for the business traveller who may have to take some mega-important decision whilst under the befuddling influence of jet-lag.

The effects can be minimised, although not entirely prevented, by adopting the mealtimes and sleep-wake times of the destination country as soon as you arrive, or even on the flight there. Be careful to avoid caffeine-containing drinks, such as coffee or tea, too close to bedtime in the destination country. Use an alarm clock to wake yourself up next morning if necessary. Punctuate the following day with your usual rituals – breakfast, morning coffee, lunch, afternoon tea, etc – to persuade your body/brain clock to make the switch to 'new' time. Go to the lavatory at your usual time of day too.

It usually takes about three or four days to get over jet-lag. The more time zones crossed, the tougher it is.

When you get back

- If you were taking malaria tablets whilst abroad, keep taking them for another *month* after returning.
- If you become ill, particularly with fever or diarrhoea, tell your doctor which countries you've visited.
- Even if you're feeling well, always consult your doctor or clinic if you were bitten by an animal or risked catching a sexually transmitted disease.

BODY MAINTENANCE

SKIN

We're born with soft, smooth, delicate skin which, throughout childhood, despite the usual quota of cuts and grazes, fares remarkably well. Young skin, with its enviable powers of regeneration, shrugs off these insults almost overnight.

But as time goes by, our skin's vitality slowly and inexorably diminishes. The youthful sheen fades, the elasticity sags, the wrinkles and blemishes accumulate.

Can these ageing effects be slowed down? Will feeding the skin with 'nutrients' help? How can we keep our skin healthy?

The ravages of time

The bad news is that, despite the millions spent on research into skin ageing by the cosmetics industry, there's no way that our skin can stay younger longer – apart from avoiding the long-term damage inflicted by the sun and cigarette smoke.

So-called skin 'nutrients' make not a jot of difference. The only effective way of feeding the skin is by feeding yourself a healthy diet (see Chapter 2), especially fruit and vegetables containing Vitamins A, C and E. There's mounting evidence that these vitamins act as anti-oxidants, mopping up destructive 'free radicals' throughout the body.

Sun damage

The risk of malignant melanoma cancer caused by over-exposure to the sun is covered on pages 141–2. This form of skin cancer is caused mainly by too much UVB, the burning ultraviolet rays that can be filtered out by sunscreens. But, there are other ultraviolet rays which most sunscreens let through. These are the UVA rays, which stimulate the pigment cells to bring on a tan. Unfortunately, a tan is not a sign of vibrant health. It's the skin's attempt at protecting itself from UV damage – and it never quite succeeds. Enough UVA rays get through to thicken the epidermis, making it leathery, to increase its cell turnover, causing pigmented blemishes such as cafe-au-lait spots, and to destroy hydrogen bonds, weakening the connective protein collagen.

The result is sags, wrinkles and blotches. In other words, too much sun speeds up ageing. After a few decades, it can also cause non-melanoma skin cancer, the second most common cancer after lung and breast. Sad, but true.

... and cigarette smoke?

Yes, this too is thought to speed up skin ageing. Studies have suggested that benzene-related chemicals in the microscopic droplets of tar floating in cigarette smoke, also destroy hydrogen bonds and weaken collagen.

Skin care

Apart from sun and smoke, the main everyday threats to skin health are excessive drying and chapping, allergies and acne.

Drying and chapping can be prevented by avoiding harsh soap, using a moisturiser and keeping out of strong dry winds. Use a mild soap, such as baby soap, or no soap at all. An ordinary moisturiser, by adding a little oil to the outer epidermis, will waterproof it and cut down evaporation.

Allergies to such things as nickel, chrome, or certain plants, can cause dermatitis or eczema. Again, apart from avoiding the allergen, a moisturiser can help, perhaps in the form of a bath oil.

Acne

Amazingly, despite the marvels of modern science, acne still can't be cured. But, with proper self-care or medical treatment, it can at least be controlled.

It happens because of androgens – sex hormones that stimulate the oil-glands and thicken the epidermis, particularly on the face, shoulders, back and chest. This sets up the chain reaction that so often leads to acne.

Each oil-gland is situated deep within a hair-root pore which soon fills with greasy gunge. This becomes hardened into a plug at the skin surface, where exposure to the air turns it dark brown – the all-too-familiar 'blackhead'. The more gunge that builds up, the bigger the blackhead.

Enter Proprionibacterium acnes. This normally friendly bacterium lives harmlessly on the skin surface, deriving nutrients from skin-oil. But if it gets into a gunge-packed pore, it wreaks havoc, multiplying like mad and producing highly irritant substances which, when they leak into the surrounding skin tissue, cause inflammation. In other words, a classic acne spot.

Cross-section of skin and hair

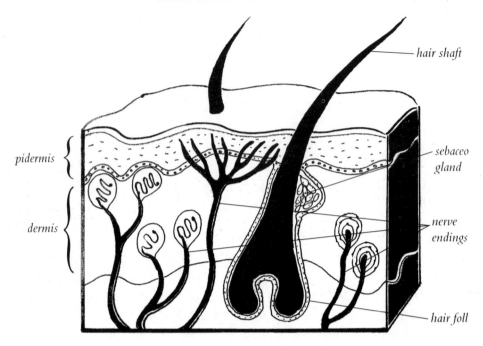

hair shaft

pidermis

sebaceo
gland

dermis

nerve
endings

hair foll

Who gets acne?

- Boys, with their higher androgen levels, are more vulnerable than girls.
- Many girls get spots in the week or two before their period, when fluid retention in the skin makes the pores more likely to clog.
- Certain types of contraceptive Pill can increase acne.
- Irregular sleep seems to make it worse.
- There's no firm evidence that chocolate causes acne.
- Acne often lingers on into the twenties, thirties and even later.
- The tendency to severe or prolonged acne seems to run in families.
- Acne is *not* caused by having a dirty skin, and is *not* infectious in any way.

What can be done about it?

You can help to keep spots at bay by avoiding harsh soaps and spirit-based astringents or face-fresheners which, although they 'cleanse' oily skin, make it react by becoming even oilier. It's also sensible to avoid greasy make-up. Instead, try the daily anti-spot routine below.

Anti-spot routine

- Wash your face twice a day with warm water.
- Each evening, give yourself a quick facial sauna by resting a hot, clean flannel over your face for a minute or two to soften the skin and open the pores.
- Follow that with a massage using clean tissues folded into a pad, working in small circles over the spot-prone area.

There are various antiseptic lotions, creams and gels which can help to control mild acne by discouraging skin bacteria – but because they don't penetrate the pores very well they may not be the complete answer. Those containing benzoyl peroxide are the most effective.

Sunlight (or UV light) is usually beneficial – perhaps by discouraging skin bacteria and promoting skin turnover. However, you should avoid oily sun-protection creams and cosmetics.

Despite the lack of scientific evidence, you may find that cutting out chocolate, cheese or some other food substance helps your skin. It's also important to eat plenty of carrots and leafy vegetables containing Vitamin A, vital for skin health. And if you've noticed your skin getting greasier after late nights, try to keep to more regular sleeping hours.

If simple self-help is not controlling the problem, your doctor might consider prescribing a long course of antibiotics to inhibit the bacteria in the pores. Alternatively, you might be referred to a dermatologist.

HEALTHY HAIR

It's as dead as a dodo, and yet it matters so much to us. We may have too little, or too much in the wrong places. It may be too greasy, or too dry. It may be sprinkled with dandruff, or plagued with headlice.

How can we keep our hair healthy?

Hair loss

We all lose hair all the time. Our hair is constantly being replaced, and it's perfectly normal to lose up to about 100 hairs a day as they reach the end of their active growth.

Each hair lasts for an average of three or four years before its follicle (root) enters a resting phase. After about three months it starts growing again.

During the resting phase the old hair is detached from the base of the follicle, and can easily be pulled out by brushing, combing or washing.

All this is perfectly normal. But sometimes the follicle can go into a different mode and, instead of making a thick, strong hair, it produces a soft, downy 'baby' hair instead. This is what happens with abnormal hair loss. The bald or thin areas are actually covered with as many hairs as before – but unfortunately they are baby hairs, and virtually invisible.

Why does it happen?

There are many possible causes – but the commonest factor is age. We all have most hair in our teens and early twenties, and then start to lose it.

In men, the hair loss occurs in patches, and follows a classic pattern – receding temples and an ever-increasing bald pate. The age at which this occurs is determined entirely by the man's inherited genes, and has nothing to do with either his 'virility' or intellect.

In women, hair loss is usually diffuse – an even thinning over the whole head. It's a very gradual process to start with, but speeds up alarmingly during and after the menopause, when the female hormones subside.

Various factors can bring on sudden hair loss. Childbirth, for example, can result in major thinning or even complete baldness in some women, as the body's immune system readjusts. Fortunately, this dire state of affairs is only temporary, and the hair grows back over the next six months or so.

Another common cause is an under-active thyroid gland. This occurs mostly in middle-aged women, and is linked to an increase in weight, a roughening of the voice, and a general slowing down physically and mentally.

Emotional shock can occasionally make someone lose their hair 'overnight' – again usually only temporarily.

Some forms of drug treatment for cancer (chemotherapy) have a similar effect. And various other illnesses and nutritional deficiency states can cause diffuse hair loss.

But most cases of patchy hair loss in women (alopecia areata) have no known cause.

What's the treatment?

Scientists have been trying to find a cure for baldness for centuries – with no real success.

If the hair loss has a medical cause, such as an under-active thyroid gland, then treatment of that condition will restore hair growth.

But if the cause is male-pattern baldness, post-menopausal thinning, or alopecia areata, then little can be done to improve things.

Hormone replacement therapy can help some women with general thinning of the hair, but by no means all. Steroid injections have been used successfully to treat alopecia areata.

But male baldness refuses to respond to virtually all the lotions and potions that have been devised to treat it.

One medication, minoxidil, does have a useful growth-stimulating effect – but in most men who've tried it the result is disappointing for the cost involved. What's more, the effect doesn't last, and if the drug is stopped, the baldness returns.

So, what can be done to help?

The answer is to make the most of what you've got.

For women, careful hair styling can usually disguise the thinning. But for men, it's mainly a matter of accepting the situation.

A hair-piece, perhaps woven into existing hair, can transform the appearance. But hair transplants, in which tiny patches of hair are transferred from the sides of the head to the hairline or crown, tend to be disappointing, unless used as a foundation for a permanent hair-piece.

Excess hair

So many women have so much hair in so many places where they don't want it, that the business of getting rid of it is worth millions. Bathrooms echo with the ooohs and ouches of plucked eyebrows, nicked legs and waxed bikini lines.

But not only is unwanted hair a cosmetic chore – it's often the cause of a great deal of real embarrassment and misery.

Our body hair pattern is mainly inherited, although in occasional cases it's altered by a hormonal disturbance. Excess hair mainly appears on the belly and thighs, the legs and arms, and the lips and nipples. Oilier skins tend to have more active hair growth. Hair colour plays a part too – darker hairs are more visible.

Women of Afro-Caribbean stock tend to have less than average body hair, whilst those of Eastern Mediterranean descent have more.

The notion that shaving, plucking or waxing stimulate hair growth is a complete myth.

Which methods are best?

It depends on practical factors like how much hair you're trying to remove, whereabouts it is, and how much time, trouble or cash you're prepared to spend.

With large areas, such as legs or arms, shaving is the most popular method for legs – quick, painless and cheap. But the sharp stubble soon returns. Creams, sprays and lotions work by weakening the hairs so that they can be washed or towelled off. But they are fairly caustic and have to be used strictly according to the makers' instructions. Many skins are too sensitive for them, or even allergic.

Waxing has the advantage of pulling the hairs out at the roots, so that new hairs take weeks to regrow. But the technique can be fiddly, rather painful, and you have to let your hairs grow long enough for the wax to get a grip.

With abrasion, you simply rub the hairs off with a pumice stone, rough mitts or oatmeal paste. Again, not suitable for delicate skins. Bleaching renders dark hairs less noticeable.

What about facial hair?

Apart from eyebrow plucking – simple and effective – or bleaching of a fuzzy upper lip, the best treatment may well be electrolysis. This uses a very fine electrical probe, itself not much thicker than a hair, to destroy each individual hair root permanently.

In trained, qualified hands electrolysis is safe and no more than a little uncomfortable. But it's a slow process and, for strongly growing hair, may need two or three attempts for each root.

Headlice

They're wingless insects about two millimetres long, with six strong hooked legs for gripping hairs, and a bellyful of human blood that they've sucked. Nits are their whitish eggs, stuck firmly to the hairs.

Contrary to popular belief, lice can't jump or fly. To get from one head to another, there must be close head-to-head contact for a few seconds. The adult louse takes the opportunity to find a fresh breeding ground.

Young children are much more susceptible because their heads are always touching each other. Their scalp skin is also thinner and easier for the lice to feed from. Clean hair is just as likely to attract lice as dirty hair. They're not spread on combs or brushes.

How can they be detected?

Itching is the big clue – but the lice may have been on the child's head for up to two months before the itching begins. Another clue is to look for the tell-tale nits. Use a special nit-comb from the chemists – they come free with

155

headlouse lotion. Some schools give them out as part of a local headlouse erad-ication campaign.

How can you get rid of headlice?

You have to use a special insecticide lotion or shampoo. Ask your pharmacist for advice. The most important thing is to make sure that every member of the family in close contact with the child has the treatment – grown-ups included.

EYES RIGHT

Considering how vulnerable they seem, our eyes are well adapted to looking after themselves. Each eyeball sits in a bony socket, protected by the brow and cheekbone, and cushioned on a pad of fatty tissue. The eyelashes catch dust and dirt, and the eyelids constantly blink to sweep antibacterial tear-fluid across the front of the eyeball. The skin of the eyelids, the thinnest in the entire body, is richly supplied with oil-glands to keep them soft and supple.

The inner surface of the eyelids and the front surface of the eyeball are covered with a membrane called the conjunctiva. This contains blood vessels which, as well as helping to supply the eye with nutrients and oxygen, bring white blood cells and antibodies to fight off bacteria and viruses. These blood vessels expand and become more visible if the conjunctiva gets inflamed (conjunctivitis or 'pink eye'). At the base of each eyelid the fold of the conjunctiva forms a continuous pocket, making it impossible for foreign bodies, such as a contact lens, to slip round behind the eyeball.

Eye-care

What should we be doing to keep our eyes shiny and bright? Surprisingly, apart from an ordinary face-wash each morning, and, if necessary, removal of make-up each evening, there's really nothing to do. Our eyes do the regular maintenance work for us. No additional help is needed. All those eye-care solutions and drops are just so much eye-wash.

Tired red eyes?

What about tea-bags or slices of cucumber for tired red eyes? Again, according to the experts, these achieve no more than if you were simply to lie back with your eyes closed and let the tear-fluid do its work. If the cucumber is taken straight from the fridge and thick-sliced, its coolness may help to constrict the blood vessels in the conjunctiva, diminishing the redness – but this effect will last just about long enough for you to look in the mirror before the vessels dilate again.

The way to prevent tired red eyes is to keep out of smokey atmospheres, go easy with alcohol (it slows your blink-rate), get more sleep, and avoid 'eye-strain'.

Eye-strain

Do your eyes ache after a day on the beach? Or when you've been reading in poor light? Does watching the television or a computer screen make them hurt? Or long hours driving? These are just a few of the many causes of eye-strain – a nasty ache behind the eyes, and sometimes the crown of the head.

But, surprisingly, what we call 'eye-strain' has nothing to do with straining the eyes. It's a pain that results from excessive clenching of muscles – but the muscles are those of the face rather than the eyes themselves.

For example, if you're out in the bright sun without sunglasses, the natural reaction is to scowl or screw your eyes up in an effort to reduce the glare. This means you're contracting the facial muscles that surround your eyes, and after a while they may start to ache.

Similarly, if you're at your desktop and you can't see the screen very clearly, it's natural to screw your eyes up in an effort to improve your focus. But, again, this clenches the facial muscles around your eyes, and before long they'll start aching.

Although there are special muscles inside each eyeball that focus the lens and adjust the iris (controlling the amount of light entering the eye), these are designed to be constantly active and do not tire or become strained like other muscles. Neither, it seems, do the tiny muscles of the eye-socket, whose job it is to make the eyes look up, down, to one side or the other or to converge on close objects. You can spend all day doing really close work and, providing you're not squinting or screwing your eyes up, you shouldn't get eye-strain.

What can you do to relieve eye-strain? A simple painkiller such as soluble aspirin, paracetamol or ibuprofen will quickly dispel the pain. A cold compress on the forehead helps too – try a packet of frozen peas in a hanky.

157

How to avoid eye-strain

To avoid eye-strain here are some simple guidleines. First, if you can't see things crystal clearly, go to your high street optometrist (optician) and make an appointment to have your eyes tested. You may need glasses or contact lenses. This is especially likely if you're in your mid-forties, when the focusing power of your natural lenses changes and you find you have more and more difficulty reading or seeing close objects clearly. If you already wear glasses or contact lenses, they may need changing to a different prescription (focusing strength).

Make sure you do actually use your glasses or lenses for such activities as reading, watching television, word processing or driving. Check that your lighting arrangements are adequate. Ideally, for reading and other close work, you need a light shining from over one shoulder.

In bright sunlight, always wear sunglasses. Polarised sunglasses are best for reducing glare, especially that reflected off the sea, sand, road, pavement or car bonnet.

Try to have a break from any job requiring concentrated visual attention, such as driving, for at least a few minutes every two hours. Take off your specs, shut your eyes or just gaze into the far distance away from the sun. This will help to relax your clenched facial muscles, and fend off any eye-strain.

How to care for your eyes
- Avoid rubbing your eyes – you might introduce infection, and if a speck of grit is there, you might scratch your eyeball.
- Always wear protective glasses or goggles if you're handling caustic chemicals or machinery that kicks up particles.
- Wear dark glasses or a wide-brimmed hat in very bright conditions.
- Be scrupulously hygienic with contact lenses – disposables are safest.
- Have your eyes checked by an optometrist every two years, and more often if you're over forty, or have high blood pressure, diabetes or a close relative with glaucoma.

EARS AND HEARING

As with our eyes, our ears need little attention to keep them in good health. Apart from washing with soap and water, it's best to leave your ears alone. You should certainly not attempt to clean your ear-holes with cotton buds or the corners of towels.

The main threats to our ears are noise, which can cause hearing loss, and infection, which can lead to much pain and irritation.

Noise exposure

Behind our ear-drums are delicate hearing organs that amplify sound and convert it to nerve signals to the brain. Although the amplification system has an inbuilt mechanism for protecting the hearing organ against loud sounds, it can't cope with the literally deafening noise produced by such things as pneumatic drills, explosions, rock concerts, and steelmaking.

Repeated or prolonged exposure to noise destroys the sensory cells in the inner ear, particularly at the higher frequencies, most important for hearing speech. The result is high-tone deafness and, in some, cases tinnitus, a ringing or buzzing in the ears.

There are particular dangers for workers in heavy industry, although the full effects may not be apparent for many years. Where the noise level exceeds 90 decibels (equivalent to an unbaffled pneumatic drill at five metres), ear protectors should be worn at all times. As a rough guide, if the prevailing noise is so loud that you can't hear yourself speak without having to shout, then you must have ear-protection.

Another noise danger, particularly worrying for young people, is the powerful amplification at heavy rock concerts, or even listening to loud music through headphones. Again, too much of this, and the result is hearing difficulty from a young age.

How loud is noise?	
Ticking watch next to ear	30 decibels
Normal conversation	60 decibels
Loud music	90 decibels
Pneumatic drill at 1 metre	120 decibels
Jet engine at 30 metres	130 decibels

Ear-wax

Wax is secreted by the lining of the ear-hole, and its main job is to work its way very slowly out of the ear, carrying dust, dirt and other detritus with it. Its other job is to repel moisture and discourage bacteria and fungi.

Normally wax is soft. But in some people, particularly older people, it becomes hardened and dry. This irritates the ear-canal – 'ear-hole', causing the person to stick their little finger in their ear to relieve the itch. This pushes the wax deep into the ear where it gets impacted and stuck. The result is temporary deafness and continued irritation.

Impacted wax can be softened with warm olive oil drops, repeated daily. If necessary, your doctor or practice nurse may remove the wax by syringing it out with warm sodium bicarbonate solution.

Ear-infection

By far the commonest type is infection of the middle ear chamber – acute otitis media. This chamber is a small air-filled space on the inner side of the eardrum in each ear. It contains the ossicles – tiny bones that amplify the sound waves and transmit them to the sense organ in the inner ear. The air in the chamber comes via a narrow duct (Eustachian tube) from the nasal cavity where the back of the nose joins the throat. Infection from a bad cold or catarrh can all too easily pass along the tube to the middle ear, especially in children.

The infected middle ear chamber becomes inflamed and filled with pus – with throbbing pain, partial deafness and usually a high temperature. If left untreated, the pus builds up into an abscess which eventually bursts through the eardrum.

If you suspect middle ear infection, you should seek medical attention without delay. Antibiotics are needed, and the sooner the better – otherwise there's a risk of long term hearing loss. In the mean time you can soothe the ear by taking a pain-killer such as paracetamol.

Another common cause is otitis externa – infection of the outer ear-canal or (ear-hole). This gives rise to intense irritation and a sharper, more stinging pain, usually accompanied by a smelly discharge. The ear itself can be extremely tender. The condition is caused by viruses, bacteria or fungi, and is often picked up from shared towels. Among older people, hardened earwax may block the ear-hole and act as a focus for irritation and infection.

Infections of the outer ear sometimes clear up on their own, but usually need antibiotic or antifungal ear-drops. Never poke anything into the ear-hole in an attempt to clean away the discharge – although a wipe with a wisp of cotton wool is OK as long as you wash your hands afterwards to avoid spreading the infection to the other ear.

What is 'glue ear'?

This is a common condition in young children in which a sticky fluid collects in the middle ear chamber and may result in hearing difficulty, especially for the spoken word. It's caused by blockage of the Eustachian tube, usually because of enlarged adenoids.

If you suspect that your child may have glue ear, then ask the doctor about a hearing test. Grommets, tiny plastic ventilation ducts inserted in the ear-drums, may be recommended, although there's some controversy about their effectiveness.

TEETH AND GUMS

Now here are parts of the body that certainly do need constant maintenance. Cleaning your teeth is a real chore, but, as everyone knows, it's crucial if you want to keep them. Two decades or so ago, in Britain, nearly four out of ten adults had no natural teeth whatsoever. Today the number of toothless adults has been halved. Tooth decay in children has improved even more rapidly, halved over the past ten years.

Why these dramatic improvements? The evidence points mainly to the advent of fluoride toothpaste and advances in dentistry. Fluoride helps to protect against tooth decay by strengthening tooth enamel and making it more acid-resistant. Regular dental check-ups, improved dental hygiene and more effective conservative dentistry have helped in the constant fight against gum disease.

Tooth decay

This is mainly a problem in childhood, although, with more elderly people retaining their teeth, it's becoming quite a problem in later life too.

The enemy is dental plaque – a sticky yellowish coating that forms on the teeth, especially in the nooks and crannies. Plaque consists of zillions of bacteria, normal inhabitants of the mouth, which multiply like crazy, feeding on the sugary residues left in the mouth after eating or drinking many sweet things.

Apart from looking and smelling rather unpleasant, the real problem with plaque is its propensity for producing acid, which starts to dissolve the tooth enamel within seconds of coming into contact with sugar residues, and continues for twenty to thirty minutes afterwards, until neutralised by the saliva.

The problem is not so much the quantity of sugar passing through the mouth, but how often it does so. Each time anything sugary is eaten or drunk the acid level is bumped up for perhaps half an hour, etching away at the tooth enamel.

Part of the answer, needless to say, is to eat or drink sugary things less often – not so easy for the average child bombarded with adverts for sweets and soft drinks. The other important defence is to brush twice daily with fluoride toothpaste, and to have regular dental check-ups. In areas where the water is fluoridated, tooth decay in children has been halved.

Gum disease

Incredible though it may seem, as many as nine out of ten adults have gum disease. What's more, the most common form, gingivitis, can eventually be much more of a threat to your teeth than the occasional cavity appearing in childhood.

The stages of gum disease

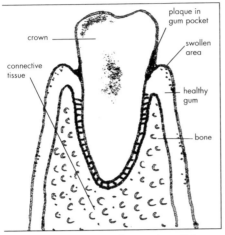

1 *Plaque encourages inflammation of the gums, which bleed during brushing*

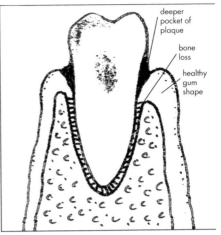

2 *The gum pocket gets deeper, as bone and tissue holding the tooth are destroyed by build-up of plaque*

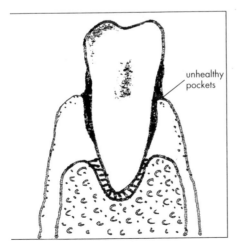

3 *The gum shrinks and the tooth looks longer. The tooth is now looser*

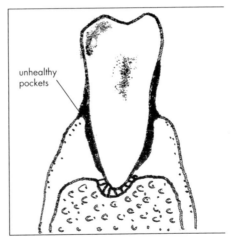

4 *Most of the bone is by now gone. The tooth will be painful, loose and will probably be lost*

The early warning sign is bleeding gums when you use a toothbrush. This happens because the gum margin around the teeth is slightly inflamed and swollen (gingivitis) thanks to irritants produced by dental plaque. The little inlets of gum between the teeth are especially vulnerable.

Sadly, all too often this apparently minor symptom is ignored – but slowly and surely the gingivitis gets steadily worse. Very soon it causes a pocket to open between the gum and the tooth. This allows the inflammation to spread deeper, destroying the fibres that anchor the tooth to the gum, making the gum recede.

Eventually, the inflammation may reach the bony socket in the jaw where it does its worst mischief either by destroying the tooth's main anchorage, or by causing an abscess or gumboil. Either way, the tooth is likely to be lost.

In some cases, gingivitis can become quite severe long before these changes have taken place. Women who are pregnant or on the Pill often suffer from very tender, bleeding gums. In some cases of acute gingivitis there may be pus oozing from the gum pockets, tainting the breath with a foul rotting odour.

You can stop gum disease in its tracks if you know how to clean your teeth carefully (see box).

How to clean your teeth properly

- Firstly, brush them carefully. Not by scrubbing hard, but with small, back-and-forth movements.
- Use a small-headed, medium-tufted toothbrush and a pea-sized dollop of fluoride toothpaste.
- Angle the brush so that you gently shift all the plaque from around the gum margins, especially on the insides of the teeth.
- Finally, tackle the surfaces between the teeth, using dental floss. It's a bit fiddly at first, but you'll soon get the hang of it – and there's no better way of reaching the plaque in the pockets beneath the gum margins.

The other important element of your gum maintenance programme should be a regular visit to your dentist or dental hygienist for a check-up and a descale and polish. Once every six months is best in order to prevent calculus (calcified plaque) building up in the gum pockets.

With this sort of care it is possible to put a stop to gum disease and give your teeth a much better chance of staying sparkling well into your twilight years.

How to floss your teeth

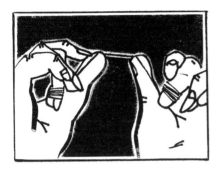

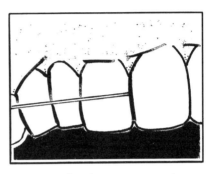

1 Wind the ends round your second fingers

2 Slip the floss between your teeth

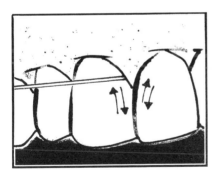

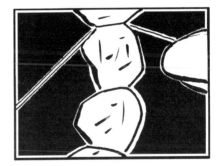

3 Ease it gently into the gum margin and out again

4 Repeat between all the teeth. Do not saw back and forth

NECK AND BACK

The human spine is a remarkable piece of engineering in the way it combines strength and flexibility. It has to be strong enough to provide a firm 'keel' for all the body's bits and pieces – but also flexible enough to allow the incredible range of movement an active person needs.

There are about 50 bones, 100 joints, 1,000 muscles and ligaments and a million nerve fibres in your neck and back. The forces generated by the muscles, the strain on the ligaments, and the pressures that develop between the bones are enormous. It's hardly surprising that things get injured or go wrong, and that spinal pain, neck pain or back ache, is one of the commonest of human afflictions.

Rear view of spine

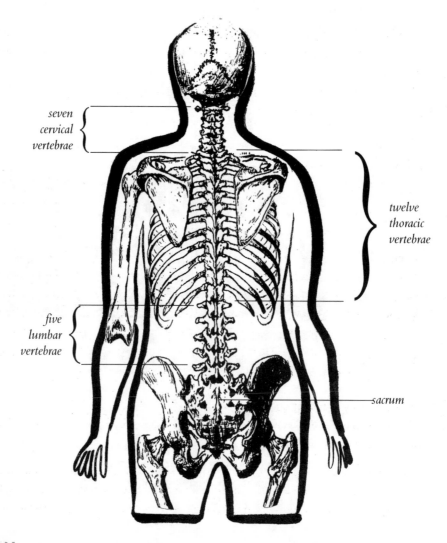

seven
cervical
vertebrae

twelve
thoracic
vertebrae

five
lumbar
vertebrae

sacrum

Neck pain

Most of the problems in the neck are muscular. The head is a surprisingly heavy item, balanced on top of a very slender column of cervical vertebrae. It's held there by ligaments and muscles, and the latter spend most of the day clenched hard, trying to keep the head erect and pointing in the right direction.

These powerful forces create tender knots in the neck muscles – trigger points of pain that used to be referred to as 'fibrositis'. Sedentary workers are especially prone to neck ache as they sit all day with their head tipped forwards, and their neck muscles rigid with painful tension.

Relief can be obtained by doing gentle stretching exercises for the neck and shoulder, and, if possible, having someone massage the tense and tender muscles.

The problem can be prevented by paying attention to posture, and making sure that desks, screens and working surfaces are at the right height.

Two other common causes of neck pain are: the so-called 'whiplash' injury, in which the neck is severely wrenched, typically in a car crash; and cervical spondylosis, wear and tear of the spinal joints as a result of degenerative changes, especially in older people. Both of these conditions can be helped with physio-therapy or osteopathy.

Back pain

One adult in five has backache – many quite severely. By far the commonest cause is a pulled muscle or a strained ligament in the small of the back. When you think how heavy the upper half of your body is, you can imagine how extreme the forces are on your lower spine, especially when you bend to lift a heavy object. If these forces are too great, or too sudden, then you'll either pull something in your back – or slip a disc.

What exactly is a slipped disc?

The discs between the vertebrae act like heavy-duty cushions, giving the spine its flexibility and resilience.

Each disc consists of a tough fibrous outer layer surrounding a soft jelly-like centre. Whenever you stand, sit, bend or lift something the pressure on the soft centres of the lumbar discs can be immense. If it's too much, the jelly bursts out of the fibrous layer and bulges into the spinal channel containing the main nerve roots to the lower back and legs. This bulge is a 'slipped disc', and if it squeezes a nerve root the result is pain in the lower back or down the leg (sciatica).

Who's most at risk?

For women the most vulnerable times are during late pregnancy, when the baby is adding to the back-strain and the ligaments are temporarily weakened; when looking after toddlers – all that lifting in and out of buggies, cot-beds and car-seats; doing the family shopping – humping heavy bags or loading the hatch-back; and after the menopause when the bones and ligaments can all too easily lose their strength.

In general, the risk is higher for people who spend all day sitting in an office, but then attack the garden or shift furniture when they get home – their backs simply aren't prepared for the extra strain. Another vulnerable group includes people employed in very heavy work, such as labourers, removal people, or steelworkers. Most vulnerable of all are long-distance delivery people who have the worst of both worlds – sitting down for hours on end, and carrying lots of heavy goods.

We're all at risk, male or female, old or young. It only takes one silly mistake or accident – a load that's a little too heavy or bulky, an awkward stumble or fall, a sudden twist, or an ill-timed stretch – and you may be left with a dodgy back for days, weeks, months or perhaps the rest of your life.

How can it be prevented?

Bending, lifting and turning in the right way, can minimise the strain on your back.

If you have to lift a heavy object from the ground, don't bend forwards at the waist. Instead, crouch down, keeping your back straight and, holding the load as closely as possible, straighten up again.

If you have to turn to one side, holding something heavy, don't twist at the waist. Instead turn your feet.

When carrying heavy shopping or luggage, try to balance the load evenly in each hand.

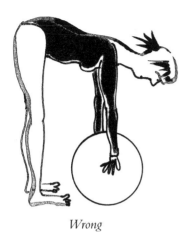
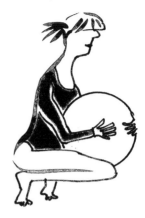

Wrong   *Right*

Bending forward for a long time – weeding the garden for instance – puts a great strain on your back. Better to get down on one or both knees.

If you spend a lot of time sitting at a desk, make sure your chair is at the right height and can swivel to avoid twisting your lumbar spine.

A lot of people get back trouble because their bed is too soft and sags in the middle. It's well worth paying extra for a more supportive mattress.

Any exercise or activity which strengthens the trunk muscles will help protect against back pain. Swimming is perhaps the best all-round form of exercise for backs.

What will relieve sudden back pain?

The first thing to do is lie flat for at least 24 hours, and then, if the pain has settled down, very carefully get to your feet. Aspirin, paracetamol or ibuprofen can be taken to start with, but not for long because the pain is a useful warning not to aggravate the problem.

If you have severe backache persisting for more than about three days, or if the pain is steadily worsening, see your doctor, or a properly qualified osteopath or chiropractor.

Ten tips for a healthy back

1 Always carry heavy loads equally in both hands.

2 Hold large objects close to your body.

3 Get a good firm grip – don't slip.

4 Keep your back straight.

5 Let your legs do the bending and turning.

6 Sit up straight – don't slouch.

7 Use a chair with a back-rest.

8 Sleep on a firm mattress.

9 Take lots of exercise – swimming's best.

10 Lose excess weight – give your back a chance.

HANDS AND FEET

Hands (and arms)

Compared with your feet, your hands have a good life. Lots of freedom, plenty of movement, a light and airy existence. And not much maintenance required, apart from some elementary manicure.

The skin of the hands may need protection against detergents, caustic substances, allergens and cold weather. Barrier cream or the right sort of gloves are usually all that's needed.

But, with more and more people using computer keyboards, a problem that is fast becoming a major threat for busy hands is RSI – Repetitive Strain Injury.

RSI

Repetitive Strain Injury is something of a catch-all term for a long list of aches and pains caused by over-using or repeatedly straining your hand, arm or shoulder. Many familiar complaints, such as tennis elbow, tenosynovitis, trigger finger, carpal tunnel syndrome, and frozen shoulder, can start this way, and could all be considered examples of RSI.

The precise symptoms depend on which part you've over-used or strained. If it's a tendon in the hand or wrist, there'll be pain and tenderness, and perhaps redness and swelling, over the injured part. Strain at the elbow causes shooting pains in the forearm, and an extremely tender spot where the tendon is attached to the elbow bone. With shoulder strain the pains may shoot down the upper arm or into the neck, and you may have great difficulty moving your arm at all – 'frozen' shoulder.

These pains are usually sharp, and made worse by doing the activity which caused them in the first place. But they may be little more than a dull ache present most of the time. They may develop gradually over months or years, or strike quite suddenly.

When you repeat a movement time and time again, for hours on end, day after day, the tendons may eventually start to show signs of wear and tear. Although they usually slide in well-lubricated sheaths and grooves, the constant rubbing and tension on them makes them slightly inflamed. This in turn makes their normally silky smooth surface a little rough – which means even more friction. A vicious circle is set up, with the pain and tenderness getting worse and worse, until that particular movement eventually becomes impossible to carry out without suffering a great deal of pain. What's more, even simple daily tasks, such as holding a toothbrush, doing up buttons, or opening tins, can become agonising. This is the typical story of tenosynovitis – tendon sheath inflammation of the wrist – a common form of RSI.

In other forms, trigger finger or thumb, the tendon becomes thickened in the friction spot, developing a little ridge which gets stuck in the groove, and then suddenly releases, like a trigger.

Sometimes the strain on the tendon in its lubricated groove forces lubricant jelly to bulge into the tissue around the tendon, creating a painless lump called a ganglion.

Tennis and golfer's elbow are rather different. With these the problem isn't so much constant rubbing of a tendon, but over-stretching of a muscle attachment to the elbow bone. Tennis elbow is an injury to the outer elbow, where the muscle which cocks the wrist is attached. Golfer's elbow is on the inner side of the elbow, at the anchorage for the muscle which flexes the wrist. You don't have to be either a tennis or golf player to suffer these injuries – you can get them lifting a heavy kettle or suitcase.

For RSI, the most vulnerable people are: keyboard operators – secretaries, telephonists, check-out persons, booking clerks, and even pianists – cleaners, hairdressers, machine operators, assembly workers, chicken packers, bank clerks, and a whole variety of sports players. Children addicted to computer games and arcade machines are frequent victims too. Some forms of RSI are regarded as industrial injuries in certain occupations, and a claim can be made for compensation.

The best treatment is rest – but it only works if you deal with the problem as soon as you start having symptoms. Tell your union safety rep if you have one, and see either the works doctor or your own GP.

Self-help for RSI

- At work, position yourself comfortably at the right height for the job, so that movements can be performed easily without strain.
- If there's any difficulty about this, seek the advice of your union safety rep.
- If equipment is stiff or substandard, again discuss it with your boss or union rep.
- If you work a keyboard, limit the number of keystrokes you make a day to 10,000 maximum.
- For highly repetitive work you should have five-minute rest-breaks every half-hour.
- If you get pains in your hand, wrist, arm or shoulder, see your doctor sooner rather than later.
- Ordinary painkillers will bring relief – but the danger is that they'll make you think you can carry on with the work, thus making the injury worse.
- The best treatment for RSI is rest.

Depending on the precise problem you might be given a cortisone injection, a splint, or an anti-inflammatory medication to take. Physiotherapy might also help. But the essence of treatment is to rest the hand or arm – which usually means changing to other duties.

Most employers are aware of the problem and are sympathetic to the need for rest. They will usually find alternative work for you. If there is difficulty with this, your union rep may be able to argue the case for you.

Healthy feet

Spare a thought for your feet – the most down-trodden part of your body. And the most put-upon. There they are, squeezed into airless shoes and stomped, pummelled and pounded all day long. In the average lifetime, they take you the equivalent of two-and-a-half times round the world. No wonder they play you up from time to time.

One of their favourite ways of complaining is by developing corns.

Corns and callouses

Corns are small, rounded hillocks of hardened, but extremely tender, skin. When our ancestors first evolved the habit of standing up on their hind legs, Nature made sure that the skin of their feet could protect itself against the skids and scuffs of everyday life. So it's specially adapted to become thick and leathery wherever it's subjected to repeated pressure or friction. This thickening is called a callous, and is not in itself painful.

But if a small area of the skin is repeatedly aggravated, a small but very thick callous develops, which then presses on the nerve-endings beneath, causing pain. This is a corn, and most of them form over a toe knuckle, where the foot is being pinched or rubbed by the shoe.

Corns are unheard of amongst Third World people who go barefoot. The soles of their feet are as thick as the soles on our shoes – but it's callous, and not corns. So, no pain.

By contrast, our feet are forced to spend most of their time in the unnatural straitjackets we call shoes – and wherever there is a pressure point, there's a risk that a corn will develop.

The crucial thing is to break the vicious cycle – pressure, thickening, corn, more pressure. It's no good reducing the corn, without dealing with the pressure that caused it in the first place.

So, first make sure that your shoes fit you properly and comfortably. Don't squeeze your toes into fashionably pointed shoes. Don't wear heels so high that your feet get crammed into the front ends. Shoes should be long enough, wide enough and – very important but often forgotten – deep enough to prevent rubbing or pinching of the toes.

If you do have a corn, or the reddened tender beginnings of one, use a ring pad around it to relieve the pressure. This has to be substantial enough to hold the shoe clear, but not so bulky that it creates more pressure elsewhere. Your chiropodist or pharmacist will advise you.

Never try to cut or pare away a corn – there's a risk that you'll introduce infection. This is particularly important for people with diabetes, who are vulnerable to festering foot problems. Gentle rubbing with a pumice stone or chiropody sponge in the bath may help a shallow corn, but is just as likely to stimulate even more thickening.

Corn plasters and corn solvent may also help to remove hardened skin – but are generally best avoided because the acid they contain can damage healthy skin (again risking infection) and will also stimulate thickening in the long run.

The surest and safest way to deal with corns is to have them treated by a qualified chiropodist. This is especially important for elderly people and those with diabetes.

Basic foot care

- Wash them daily with warm soapy water and dry well between the toes.
- Change tights and socks daily. Men, this means you too.
- Go barefoot as much as possible – but wash your feet first!
- Cut toenails straight across. This helps to prevent ingrowing toenails.
- Make sure your shoes fit you properly, especially across the instep and at the toes.

Athlete's foot

This extremely common fungal infection causes itching, soreness, redness, and mushy or flaky peeling between the toes, and sometimes spreading onto the instep or sole of the foot. In some cases the fungus infects the nails, making them discoloured and separate from the nailbed.

The spaces between the toes are perfect for the fungus. An abundance of sweat glands and decaying discarded skin cells means that they're like hot steamy jungles with plenty of 'compost' to provide a breeding ground.

Athlete's foot is easily picked up anywhere warm and damp where people go barefoot. The changing-room floor, the pool-side, the games mat, are all classic pick-up places. But many people catch it at home – by sharing towels or flannels, or from the bathmat or bathroom floor. In other words, one member of the family brings the fungus home, and it quickly spreads to the rest.

Here's how to tackle it.

First, keep your feet as dry as possible to discourage the spread of the fungus. This means either wearing shoes that let your feet 'breathe' – made of a natural material, such as leather, rather than synthetic – or open sandals rather than tight lace-ups.

The same goes for tights or socks – none if you can get away with it. The hotter the weather, and the sweatier your feet, the more important it is to keep them well ventilated.

Second, bathe your feet daily in cool soapy water, and dry thoroughly, especially between the toes, preferably with disposable tissues to avoid spreading the fungus to the rest of the family. It's also important to use a separate bath-mat.

After drying, put anti-fungal talcum powder on the affected area, again especially between the toes. This can be bought over-the-counter from the chemist's. Use it liberally. Also shake it into your shoes and slippers, particularly at the toe end – and if you wear socks, into those too.

Make sure your tights and socks are clean and fresh every day, and try not to wear the same shoes two days running. Give them a chance to dry out thoroughly between times.

It's important to keep this treatment going for at least ten days after the condition seems to have cleared to ensure eradication of the fungus – otherwise it'll soon start niggling again.

Many people find that surgical spirit, dabbed between the toes after bathing, clears athlete's foot quite quickly, and can also prevent it returning.

If these simple measures don't control it for you, especially if it's spreading, seek your doctor's advice. New treatments are available which can eradicate it in a short time.

LATER LIFE

Most of the advice in this book applies just as much to older people as it does to those under sixty. The basic principles of healthy eating, keeping active, feeling good, enjoying sex, travelling well, and maintaining your bodywork are just as important for getting the best out of later life as they are for younger people.

But, having said that, the changes that ageing brings about, and the new demands of retirement, or perhaps of living alone, present special challenges for older people.

This chapter looks at some of the main aspects of good health for the over-sixties and how you can not only add years to your life, but also life to your years.

A NEW BEGINNING

There are many positive things about reaching what has been described as 'the third age' of life. You've been through the impetuosity and inexperience of youth; the maturity and responsibility of your middle years; and now you've entered the more relaxed and reflective phase of your life in which you not only have the wisdom to know what you enjoy doing, but also the time in which to do it.

It is a great opportunity. After a lifetime of working for others, perhaps in quite a narrow field, you can now branch out and develop all sorts of interests and talents that have lain undiscovered or untapped within you. You can discover aspects of yourself that you'd forgotten you had, and you can share them with your partner, family and friends. Far from being the closing of doors, this time of your life can mark a new beginning.

Keeping involved

It's important not to think that, just because you've retired, you no longer have any contribution to make – that you now have to move over to make way for the young ones. There is still a great deal to be done if you're prepared to do it, and many ways you can continue to use your skills and experience, perhaps part-time (or even full-time) employment, voluntary work, a course of study, community groups, training young people, leisure activities – the choice of opportunities today is wider than ever. Nor need physical incapacity be so much of a problem these days, with phones, faxes, computers and other new technology tumbling down in price to help you communicate with family, friends and colleagues.

Decisions, decisions

Deciding which of the many possibilities to take up may be the most difficult thing. Perhaps it might be easier if you ask yourself a few basic questions:

A few basic questions
- **Do I need to keep working for the money?**
- **Or do I want to work for the satisfaction of having a job?**
- **Do I have skills or interests I'd like to develop?**
- **Are there particular people I'd like to help or devote more time to?**
- **Do I want to stay here or move somewhere else?**
- **How can I best keep myself in good health?**

The most important thing is to keep in touch with people, keep active, and keep involved. Don't let yourself drift into a state of passive detachment or isolation – so often the recipe for rapid decline.

KEEPING BODY AND SOUL TOGETHER

The best approach to keeping your body and soul in good order is to follow the advice in earlier chapters of this book. But, of course, there's no denying that age does often bring special physical and mental problems. These aren't all exclusive to older people, but they're the sorts of ailments and conditions that very commonly interfere with later life and have to be tackled and overcome in order to enjoy the best of health in old age.

HEALTHY BOWELS

Older people are more prone to certain bowel problems such as constipation and diverticular disease. Bowel habits vary greatly from person to person. Twice a day, or once a week, for example – both are 'normal' in the sense that thousands of healthy people manage perfectly well on either of these routines. Many have no routine at all – just when the mood takes them. That too is normal.

Doctors usually regard 'constipation' as difficulty or discomfort in passing stools, especially if this is different from the person's usual bowel habit.

The main cause is a lack of fibre in the diet. Fibre is the name for the unabsorbable substances in food, mostly derived from the cell walls of plants. Only partly broken down by our digestive enzymes, the fibre forms a squidgy paste which passes right through our intestines. It used to be called roughage – but perhaps 'smoothage' would be a better term because it works by softening and bulking the motions, giving the bowels something to work on.

Another common cause is 'lazy bowels' – repeatedly ignoring the feeling of wanting to go (the 'call to stool' as doctors quaintly put it), and eventually losing the bowel habit – a common problem among elderly people. Hence their widespread reliance on laxatives.

The other common bowel problem in older people is diverticular disease, a condition in which small pockets develop in the wall of the large intestine (colon) and can become inflamed. This usually causes colicky pain, and perhaps blood in the motions, as well as constipation.

Older people may also develop cancer of the bowel, the first sign of which may be constipation with or without intermittent diarrhoea. The risk of bowel cancer begins to increase over the age of about fifty. Any older person who's noticed a change in the usual bowel habit lasting more than two or three weeks should see a doctor for a check-up, just to be on the safe side.

Getting going again
- Eat more fibre. Here's how.
- Perhaps a cereal or wholemeal toast for breakfast, with a piece of fruit.
- Maybe wholemeal bread sandwiches, a jacket potato, wholewhea pasta, beans or salad for lunch – again with a piece of fruit.
- And lots of extra vegetables with your evening meal – yes, and the fruit.
- This does *not* mean you'll put on weight because, as diets like the F-Plan showed, fibre is satisfying without being loaded with calories.
- And whilst you're building up the fibre, make an effort to re-train your bowels. Never ignore the slightest 'call to stool'.
- Wean yourself off the laxatives, and spend a few minutes each day giving your bowels a chance to respond to their new challenge!

STRONGER BONES

How often do you trip on a kerb, or slip on a mat, or stumble when someone lurches into you?

If you're an older person, any one of these everyday incidents could mean a broken wrist, fractured hip or crushed spine. All too often the bones are so thin and weak that the slightest strain or impact is just too much – the result is weeks in hospital and months of disability, with a high risk of complications, such as thrombosis or pneumonia.

The main culprit is osteoporosis – a degenerative process which is an inevitable consequence of ageing. Problems are most likely in those older people whose osteoporosis is particularly severe, and whose bones have lost so much strength that they are most at risk of fractures.

The bones gradually lose their mineral content – particularly the calcium compound which gives them rigidity – a process which begins very slowly from the mid-thirties onwards and increases rapidly from the age of about fifty, especially in women, before slowing again in old age. The hormonal changes of the menopause make women particularly susceptible in middle and old age – the earlier the menopause, the greater the risk.

Osteoporosis can also be caused by rheumatoid arthritis, an overactive thyroid gland, and a number of other chronic diseases. It may also result from prolonged treatment with steroids, or from prolonged alcoholism.

What are the symptoms?

The worrying thing about osteoporosis is that there usually aren't any warning symptoms. Suddenly, you break a bone after a fall or some more trivial incident – most commonly the hip, wrist or spine – and that's that.

If the vertebrae (spinal bones) are becoming slowly crushed under your own weight, then pressure on the nerves of the back may cause nagging aches and pains from neuralgia or fibrositis.

Ordinary X-rays can only show up severe thinning of the bone. Recently it's become possible to detect very slight loss of bone density using sophisticated techniques – but unfortunately too few clinics or hospitals have the necessary equipment at present.

How can it be prevented?

It's important to have sufficient calcium in your diet. Dairy products are an excellent source – best in the form of low-fat milk and cheeses. One pint of skimmed or semi-skimmed milk a day is likely to provide all the calcium you need. Taking extra calcium as supplements won't make your bones any stronger.

It's also important to have enough vitamin D, which helps the calcium to get into the bones. Oily fish such as sardines, tuna, mackerel, herring, pilchards and salmon are very good sources, or Vitamin D can be taken as a supplement – but beware overdosing.

Regular exercise is one of the best ways of building up your bone density and strength. More-active people have thicker bones which are more resistant to osteoporosis. You don't have to become a fitness freak – just be a little more active than usual. Walk short distances instead of hopping on a bus or taking the car. Walk up stairs instead of taking the lift. Try to walk for at least ten minutes every day – and if possible get involved in some activity that's even more energetic.

Self-help for stronger bones

1. Eat a healthy balanced diet, with generous amounts of milk or cheese each day – preferably low fat.

2. Eat fish at least twice weekly – preferably oily fish.

3. Ask your pharmacist or doctor about taking extra calcium and/or Vitamin D.

4. Become more active – do a little more each day. Try to go for at least a ten-minute walk every day. Take up a physical activity you enjoy.

Mobile joints

One of the problems of getting older is getting stiffer. Often this is simply through lack of exercise – not enough activities to keep the muscles stretched and the joints supple (see Chapter 3 for guidance on this). But, in many cases, the problem is arthritis – the biggest cause of physical disability in the developed world. Arthritis is inflammation of, or damage to, the joints. There are at least a dozen different types, some more likely to cause joint damage than others. Some types affect only one or two joints – others many. Some come on suddenly – others get slowly and steadily worse. Some cause occasional 'flare-ups' which usually leave the joints a little more damaged each time.

The symptoms vary enormously, depending not only on the type of arthritis the sufferer has, but also on how badly they have it, how long it's gone on, and how well they respond to treatment.

For most sufferers, the usual symptoms are discomfort, pain, stiffness, and a lot of difficulty and frustration. But more pain doesn't necessarily mean more damage – and most cases don't result in severe disability.

The type of arthritis most often affecting older people is osteoarthritis (OA) – so-called 'wear-and-tear' arthritis, although it mainly runs in families. About one older person in three has some OA. Contrary to popular belief, it's not caused by dampness, cold or something you've eaten – although these can make the pain and stiffness worse. With OA, the cartilage covering the bone in the joint becomes worn, rough and split, and the bone-ends deformed. It often begins in the big joint at the base of the thumb, or the end joints of the fingers, making them knobbly. It also tends to affect the feet, knees, hips and the chain of tiny joints that articulate the spine. A joint injured in youth is often susceptible later on.

What can be done to help?

Most sufferers find that over-the-counter painkillers, such as soluble aspirin, paracetamol or ibuprofen, are a great help. It's also sensible to lose as much excess weight as possible, to avoid straining the joints. In general, regular exercise is important to keep muscles and ligaments toned up – gentle stretching or swimming are ideal. Heat in the form of a warm bath, heat-lamp, hot water bottle or embrocation, is particularly soothing for OA and rheumaticky aches.

Physiotherapy is important to relieve symptoms and keep joints as mobile and strong as possible. Occupational therapists can give advice on how to make day-to-day living and working more manageable and less of a strain on your joints.

In severe cases, surgery may be needed to improve the function of damaged or deformed joints. An osteoarthritic hip or knee, for example, can be replaced with an artificial one – banishing the pain and completely transforming the sufferer's life.

Cataracts

Like looking through muslin, or a smear, everything is murky, lacklustre and dull, each sparkle a haze, each detail a blur. Cataract is an eye condition in which the lens, normally as clear as crystal, becomes more and more clouded.

It's a particular problem for elderly people, affecting about one in five between sixty-five and seventy-five, and as many as half of those aged eighty.

Unfortunately, a cataract can't be helped simply by wearing glasses. The only way to deal with it is by having an operation to remove the clouded lens altogether. But the good news is that, with modern techniques, this can be done quickly and easily without the need to stay in hospital – and the improvement is nearly always dramatic.

Most cataracts happen as a result of the ageing process – a hardening of the central part of the lens, which in some older people is enough to interfere with the supply of nutrients to the clear lens cells, making them opaque. Cataract is also common in people with poorly controlled diabetes, or who are on long-term steroids.

Surprisingly, almost everyone over the age of about sixty-five has some degree of cataract – but, because it develops so slowly, and usually from the outer edge of the lens inwards, there's often little interference with vision. About one older person in four eventually has it badly enough, in one or both eyes, to need treatment.

What can be done?

The prospect for cataract sufferers has been transformed by the wonders of modern eye surgery. Not only can the opaque lens be removed, but in recent decades it has become possible to replace it with a tiny clear plastic lens implant. Whereas in the past the person would have needed strong glasses to correct for the loss of the natural lens, now, in many cases, that isn't necessary.

There are various techniques, but the commonest involves the lens implant being lodged in exactly the same place as the original lens, held there by very fine plastic stays.

The first step is to make sure the new lens is the right size and power (strength). This is achieved by taking careful measurements beforehand using special optical equipment.

The operation itself is usually performed under local anaesthetic as a 'day-case' – in and out the same day. Previously, a ten-day stay in hospital was needed. One eye is usually done at a time, the worse first.

With the help of a binocular microscope and diamond-tipped scalpel, the surgeon makes a tiny incision in the rim of the clear round 'window' of the eye (cornea), through which the old lens is removed and the new one inserted. The incision is then stitched using very fine sutures, half the diameter of a human hair.

A soft pad may be put over the eye for a day or so while the cornea begins to heal, and an eyeshield at night. Ordinary painkillers will ease any aching in the first twenty-four hours.

The difference in vision can be remarkable. Colours are vivid again, everything is brighter. Some patients may need glasses after the operation, perhaps for reading. But, with the latest techniques being developed, using bifocal implants, the patient can see sharply both near and far without further help.

Glaucoma

Glaucoma is a common and potentially blinding eye disorder, mainly affecting older people. Glaucoma has a nasty habit of creeping up on you and it runs in families.

In its usual form it causes a slow and steady build-up of fluid in the eyeballs, which presses against the retina (the light-sensitive screen) and causes patches of blindness in the field of vision. The trouble is that these blind spots can be quite large before they're noticeable, and they're permanent. But the sooner the condition is diagnosed with a simple test at the optometrist's, the sooner treatment can be started to control the fluid build-up and save the remaining vision.

Everyone who's forty or over should make sure they have a regular eye-check – especially if they have a family history of glaucoma, or an associated condition such as diabetes or high blood pressure. The eye-check is free for people with diabetes or those aged forty or over with a parent, brother, sister or child who has had glaucoma diagnosed.

Prostate problems

About three out of four men over the age of fifty will need treatment for benign prostatic hypertrophy, BPH – an enlarged prostate gland.

What is this near-universal condition? What goes wrong? And how can it be successfully treated?

Let's start with the prostate gland itself. It's a tough rubbery gland, normally about the size and shape of a chestnut, located just beneath the bladder in men. Down through the middle of the prostate runs the urethra, the outlet tube which carries urine to the penis. The gland's job is to make seminal fluid, the salty liquid that the sperms swim in during ejaculation.

In later life, the gland very gradually enlarges – a normal part of the ageing process. Problems arise if the swollen gland tissue constricts the urethra and bulges into the bladder, distorting its outlet valve.

The symptoms, very mild to begin with, can become extremely unpleasant. 'Benign' merely means non-cancerous.

What are the symptoms?
These develop very slowly over the years. One of the first to be noticed is difficulty starting to pass water, especially in the mornings – standing there waiting for something to happen. Another is weakening of the flow – as though the tap is only half turned on. Then there may be dribbling at the finish – particularly annoying because it dampens the underpants. A very common complaint is the need to go far too often, sometimes in a great hurry, combined with a feeling that the bladder hasn't fully emptied (which indeed it hasn't). Night after night may be disturbed by somnolent staggerings to the loo.

Are there any complications?
In some cases the inadequate emptying leads to repeated attacks of cystitis (bladder infection) needing antibiotic treatment. Another possible complication is acute retention, an inability to pass any water at all. This can be triggered by

a drinking binge. The bladder becomes horribly overstretched and, as you can imagine, is extremely painful.

More insidious and damaging is chronic retention in which the bladder is stretched over a period of months or years. The problem here is that the pressure may also stretch the pipes to the kidneys, eventually causing renal failure.

Finally, some cases of prostatic enlargement are *not* benign. Cancer of the prostate is the third commonest cancer in men – one reason why it's important to see the doctor sooner rather than later with prostatic symptoms.

What's the treatment?

In the first instance, medication can usually help. There are several drugs which can relax the urethra and bladder outlet, improving the urine flow. Another group of drugs reduces the size of the prostate by counteracting the effect of male hormone on the gland. Although medication can keep the urine flowing well for a while longer, many men eventually need surgery.

The usual operation is trans-urethral resection, in which a fibrescopic viewing instrument is inserted into the penis and threaded along the urethra to the prostate. There a tiny scraper is manipulated to shave off slivers from the swollen gland tissue until the urethra has been widened sufficiently.

Results are usually excellent, with a major improvement of symptoms. Apart from a few weeks of blood in the urine, there are very few side effects. Sexual orgasm in particular is usually unaffected, although some men become impotent. However, orgasm doesn't produce ejaculation from the penis because it shoots into the bladder instead. So men who wish to father children should have their semen stored before the operation for future artificial insemination.

Other types of operation may be performed according to circumstances, especially the size of the gland. Newer techniques involving microwaves and lasers to widen the bladder outlet show great promise, but are still waiting to be properly tested.

Self-help for your prostate

1. Be aware of the symptoms of BPH and see the doctor if they are bothersome.

2. Don't go on any drinking binges – you may trigger acute retention.

3. Take tablets as directed, but remember they usually only postpone surgery.

4. If you're going to have surgery and you wish to father children, ask about preserving sperm samples for artificial insemination.

5. Very small numbers of men complain of impotence after they've recovered from surgery. If you have this problem, counselling may help.

Incontinence

It's a startling fact that more than one woman in three will suffer from loss of bladder control at some time in her life – usually in later years. About one in ten has it badly enough to need to take special precautions. And it's not just a female problem – thousands of older men suffer from dribbling incontinence.

Incontinence is an involuntary or unintentional leakage of urine, from a few drops to the whole bladderful, depending on the type of incontinence.

By far the commonest type is 'stress incontinence' – nothing to do with 'stress' in the usual sense of the word, but everything to do with sudden pressure on the bladder. It's leakage, usually a small spurt, that happens with coughing, sneezing, laughing, lifting, bending or other exertion. Another common type is 'urge incontinence' – an uncontrollable need to pass water. This is usually caused by a bladder infection.

Older men with untreated prostate trouble may suffer from 'overflow incontinence' – dribbling from a chronically distended bladder that, because of obstruction, can't empty itself.

The fourth main type is caused by damage to the nerves that control the bladder, so that the whole bladder empties automatically when it's full.

What can be done to help?

You can usually do quite a lot to help yourself. As a first step you can cut down on the amount you drink, and make sure you're not too far from the nearest loo.

For stress incontinence, try doing special 'internal' exercises to strengthen your pelvic floor muscles. These are the muscles you use to stop urinating – check them out next time you go to the loo – clenching them gives you a sort of tightening feeling inside. To strengthen them you should hold them clenched for about ten seconds and then relax, repeating this ten times. Have about ten of these exercise sessions a day. Because it's invisible, you can do it almost anywhere. You should start noticing an improvement within about two weeks.

Self-help for a leaky bladder

1. Be reassured, you're not alone. About three million people in Britain have a bladder control problem.

2. Cut down on drinks, especially tea and coffee – caffeine is a diuretic.

3. If you smoke, pack it in – the less often you cough the better.

4. Never stray too far from a loo.

5. For minor stress incontinence, do pelvic floor exercises.

6. Women may also be helped by disposable vaginal bladder supports from the chemists.

7. If necessary, choose a suitable type of disposable absorbent pad.

8. Seek the advice of your doctor, local continence advisor or physiotherapist.

In addition, for women, disposable tampon-shaped bladder supports are available which can be inserted into the vagina to help prop up the sagging pelvic floor while you're waiting for the exercises to have their strengthening effect.

Another approach is to wear disposable absorbent pads or briefs. There are many types and sizes available in the chemists. If you're too embarrassed to raise the subject there, you should consult your local continence advisor or physiotherapist (you can obtain the address from your GP receptionist).

For some cases, an operation to hoist up the bladder neck is the only answer – usually done under general anaesthetic through an incision along the bikini line. Recently a 'keyhole' version of the operation, laparoscopic culposuspension, has been introduced. Not yet widely available, it's done under local anaesthetic, involves only two tiny cuts and needs a much shorter stay in hospital.

DIZZINESS AND GIDDINESS

Dizzy spells may sound rather comical, but they're not so funny for the people who keep having them – especially if they happen without warning and last more than a few seconds.

Most of us have experienced the odd time when we've suddenly felt dazed, light-headed, faint or unsteady – for instance if we've stood up quickly from a crouched position, or we've just had some awful shock. For a moment or two the lights seem to dim or we 'see stars' and have to hold on to something to steady ourselves.

But some people get dizzy spells like this much more often, more severely. Some actually faint, temporarily losing consciousness. Others become really giddy, their head in such a spin that they vomit.

What causes dizziness?

Far and away the commonest cause is some interference to the blood supply to the base of the brain. For some sufferers, standing up quickly makes the blood pressure drop for a few seconds, and this may be enough to starve the brain's circulation temporarily, causing the dizzy feeling. This is called postural hypotension, and becomes more likely as we get older. It can be a particular

problem for people whose arteries are partly clogged and whose brain circulation is less than perfect anyway. It's also a complication of diabetes and a possible
side-effect of taking blood-pressure tablets.

Another common problem, especially in older people with a touch of arthritis
in their neck, is a temporary pinching of the arteries to the base of the brain
caused by turning or leaning their head to one side.

A third problem, more common in older people, is Ménière's disease. This is a
little-understood condition which can lead not only to dizziness and giddy
turns – sometimes lasting many hours a day, for weeks, months or even years –
but also, in many cases, distressing tinnitus (ringing, buzzing, hissing or howling
in the ears) and perhaps even deafness.

What can be done for dizzy or giddy spells?

It very much depends on the cause. If you start having them for no obvious
reason, particularly if they continue for more than a few days, you should see
your doctor to try to find out why they're happening, so that the underlying
cause can be treated.

Postural hypotension can sometimes be helped by medication. So too can
certain problems with the brain's circulation. Anaemia can be treated by taking
extra iron or other food supplements. Ménière' disease can usually be greatly
helped by special medication.

VARICOSE VEINS

Varicose veins are particularly common among older people, especially women (although younger people may suffer too). They can spell years of aching discomfort and swollen feet.

They are bulging, twisted, knobbly veins on the legs, mostly on the backs of the calves or inner thighs. They bulge more when standing, and ache more towards the end of the day. They can also itch maddeningly, and make the ankles or feet swell. Hot weather aggravates them. If knocked or scratched, they may bleed profusely – perhaps badly enough to be a medical emergency. They can also lead to phlebitis and leg ulcers.

What causes them?

A combination of heredity, obesity, pregnancy and especially gravity. Varicose veins are the price some people pay for walking on two legs rather than four.

When we stand up, the blood in the veins of our legs keeps flowing upwards to the heart, thanks to special one-way valves in the deeper veins. These, plus the squeezing action of our leg muscles, counteract the effect of gravity.

If, for some reason, the valves fail, then pressure builds up in the leg veins. The deep veins are hemmed in by muscles and can't expand, but the superficial veins just under the skin can be easily overstretched. The result is those all-too-familiar dilated knobbly varicosities.

How can they be helped?

Preventing them isn't easy. If you think your veins are beginning to bulge or itch, then try to spend more time with your legs up – easier said than done! – but in the late stages of pregnancy it can certainly help.

When standing for long periods, try rocking very slightly backwards and forwards on your feet to keep your leg muscles working.

Perhaps a more practical step for most people is to wear elasticated hosiery (also known as 'graduated compression' hosiery). For women, special lycra tights and stockings are obtainable from most good pharmacies, and come in a range of attractive shades. For men, elasticated thigh-to-ankle leggings are available.

Simple varicose veins need only mild compression (5–10mmHg), more severe veins need medium compression (around 20mmHg).

What can the doctor do?

There are two main ways of dealing with severe varicose veins. First, sclerotherapy – injecting them with a fluid that shrinks them and seals them off. This can be very effective, but isn't permanent, because new veins eventually bulge.

The other treatment is an operation in which the varicose veins are disconnected from the inner deep veins and tied off with ligatures. This involves making just a few tiny incisions and can be done under local anaesthetic as a day case. Sometimes, the main varicose vein is stripped out at the same time.

After these treatments, you'll need to wear elasticated bandages or strong compression hosiery (25–30mmHg) for about six weeks, and do plenty of walking, to allow healthy veins to become established.

ALZHEIMER'S DISEASE

Alzheimer's disease is a cruel, dreadful and very sad condition. It's the commonest form of dementia, a gradual deterioration of brain function, affecting about half a million people in Britain, mostly those over sixty-five. It's also the fourth biggest killer after heart disease, cancer and stroke.

The first signs are so innocuous as to be hardly unexpected in an elderly person – increasing forgetfulness, especially for recent events, coupled with a tendency to lose track of conversations and make rather unreasonable judgments. But, after a while, more sinister symptoms appear – episodes of confusion, uncontrollable restlessness, irrational behaviour and startling swings of mood. The sufferers become more and more like a very demanding small child, only occasionally understanding what's happening to them. Eventually, their personality breaks up and even the simplest things become impossible – they can't bathe or dress themselves, feed themselves, or go to the lavatory – making them completely dependent on nursing care.

Most Alzheimer's sufferers get worse very gradually over several years. But a few deteriorate rapidly within a few months.

The usual type of Alzheimer's mainly affects the over-seventies – more often women than men. But there is a rarer type which occurs in younger people in their forties and fifties, men more than women. This type has a genetic cause and tends to run in families.

What causes it?

We know that more and more of the brain cells wither and die as the disease progresses and that the brain tissue literally shrinks. But what we don't know is why this happens. One possibility is that Alzheimer's may be caused by a dormant virus infection caught many years previously, sensitising the brain cells to eventual attack by the body's own immune system – but the evidence for this is scanty.

Another theory is that the condition is linked to chronic aluminium poisoning from tainted drinking water or food cooked in aluminium pans. Again the evidence is inconclusive. The early onset type, with one or two members of the family getting it in middle age, seems to be owing to an inherited biochemical abnormality in the brain.

Is it curable?

Sadly, no. But medication and psychotherapy can be given to alleviate the anxiety and depression, or the agitation and restlessness, that so many sufferers, and their carers, have to endure. Sleep, in particular, can usually be improved.

Carers, family and friends can help to ease the suffering by understanding the condition and maintaining as calm and well-ordered a routine as possible.

Advice and information is helpful to start with, and later community services such as home helps, district nursing, day centre care and respite care.

Eventually though, the inevitable may have to be faced, and the sufferer admitted to a nursing home or hospital for permanent full-time care.

STROKE

Do you usually think of a stroke as a sudden paralysis down one side of the body? Or sudden slurring of speech? Or sudden deterioration in normal mental functioning?

It may be any of these – or none of these. The possible consequences are many and varied, ranging from a barely noticeable temporary disturbance to a massive chronic paralysis, and perhaps death.

What goes wrong?

Like any other tissue in the body, the brain must have a good blood supply, bringing vital oxygen and nutrients. Indeed, the brain is very sensitive to a lack of blood, being permanently damaged within three or four minutes if the supply is cut off for any reason.

Each part of the brain has its own artery, dividing into smaller and smaller branches, supplying smaller and smaller areas. If the main artery or one of its branches gets blocked with a thrombosis (clot), or ruptures and bleeds, then the part of the brain it supplies will be damaged. The effects will depend on the size of the artery, the amount of damage and the function of that particular part of the brain.

What are the symptoms?

There may be paralysis – often of one side of the face or body, affecting the arm and leg. This is called hemiplegia, and is usually accompanied by numbness affecting the same side. There may be difficulty speaking or swallowing, visual disturbances, difficulty recognising or naming people or things, loss of memory, inability to think clearly, or loss of bladder or bowel control. If the vital brain stem is damaged, then breathing and perhaps even the heartbeat will stop.

How sudden is it?

Again it depends. If the cause is a cerebral thrombosis, the effects usually appear over a few hours with steadily increasing disability. With a cerebral haemorrhage the stroke is much more sudden, often with severe headache, vomiting and perhaps loss of consciousness.

How common is it?

Very – about one person in three can expect to suffer a stroke, usually in old age. About one person in seven will die from it.

Who's most vulnerable?

The older we are, the more likely we are to have a stroke. But for any given age, some people are more at risk than others.

Having high blood pressure, diabetes, high cholesterol, or a family history of strokes will all increase the risk. Strokes are more likely in the few days after a heart attack. Some people have warning signs consisting of brief lapses of normal functioning, temporary weaknesses or paralyses, known as transient ischaemic attacks.

Can a stroke be prevented?

By following the well-known advice about healthy eating, moderate drinking and giving up smoking, you'll help to reduce your risk of a stroke. The aim is to keep your blood pressure under control and prevent the build-up of the fatty deposits in the arteries which causes clogging. Many experts recommend taking half an aspirin a day to help prevent thrombosis.

What if someone has a stroke?

Call the doctor as soon as you suspect a stroke – the damage can sometimes be limited by prompt treatment.

Most sufferers are admitted to hospital – but this will depend on how severe the stroke is. Usually various tests will be done to confirm the cause and pinpoint the area of damage.

What are the chances of recovery?

Again it varies. Quite severe or even total paralysis of one side can sometimes recover within days or weeks. In other cases it takes much longer, or there may be very little improvement. In general, those functions that are likely to show the biggest gains usually start to do so within two or three weeks.

What help is available?

The community nurse will help with home nursing. The physiotherapist can advise on exercises to maintain and improve strength and flexibility. The occupational therapist teaches sufferers how to manage, and assesses the need for various devices and equipment to make life easier. The speech therapist can help the stroke sufferer to communicate.

Beating a stroke

1. To reduce your risk of a stroke, stay slim, stop smoking, drink within recommended limits, have your blood pressure checked regularly, avoid fatty foods, cut down on salt, and learn to cope with stress.

2. Many doctors recommend that people over fifty should take half a soluble aspirin a day (after a meal) to prevent thrombosis.

3. Call the doctor as soon as you suspect someone's had a stroke.

4. Be optimistic and encouraging. Depression is the biggest enemy – for carers as well as sufferers.

5. Make sure you get all the help that's available. Keep badgering if necessary.

6. Ask about grants and allowances.

7. Join the local 'stroke club' – details from your doctor or the Stroke Association.

HYPOTHERMIA

This dangerous drop in the body's 'core' temperature – the temperature of the brain, heart and blood – is a common problem we must all be alert to in frail, elderly people living alone.

Poor circulation, an under-active thyroid gland, severe arthritis, perhaps a stroke – these are all factors which may make a person hypothermic, *even in a relatively warm environment.* The body's temperature regulating system breaks down, the normal shivering response ceases, and their temperature slips to 35°C (95°F) or lower. This makes their brain slow right down, their breathing very shallow and their blood thicken. They can no longer think clearly or summon up the energy to move. The great danger is thrombosis or pneumonia.

The most important thing is to be aware of the risk, and that it doesn't have to be Arctic conditions for hypothermia to happen. Any ambient temperature below 21°C (70°F) can mean danger to someone who is susceptible.

The other point is that, because their 'body thermostat' isn't working properly, hypothermic people don't usually recognise that they're cold. Their skin might be pink and quite warm to the touch, whilst their actual core temperature is way down.

It's important for friends and neighbours to make regular visits to those at risk, and to check on heating, draughts, bedding, food and warm clothing. You may also be able to help by sorting out their heating bill and ensuring that any benefits, grants or allowances they may be entitled to are applied for.

KEEPING WARM IN WINTER

- Make sure that the room you spend most time in is warm enough. Apply for a heating allowance or other benefit if necessary.
- Get someone to help you deal with draughts. Ask your local housing department.
- Wear warm clothing. Many thin layers are better than a few thick ones. Put on a hat – one-fifth of body heat is lost through the head.
- Have several hot drinks and eat at least one hot meal a day. Ask social services for help if necessary.
- Make sure you have plenty of warm bedclothes. Wear bedsocks. Use an electric blanket, but don't forget to switch it off once you're in bed.
- Do your best to keep in touch with other people.

SAFETY AND SECURITY

Older people are more prone to accidents – particularly falls, burns and road accidents. Problems with giddiness, arthritis, poor eyesight or brittle bones may all contribute to the risk of slipping or falling. Forgetfulness and drowsiness increase the likelihood of burns. Failing sight and hearing, and a lack of mobility make older people more vulnerable to road traffic.

Because they are comparatively defenceless, older people are also often victims of muggings and break-ins.

Safety checklist for older people

- Make sure stairs and passages are well lit – there's no point in skimping on lightbulbs. If necessary, have a good torch handy.
- Put a rubber mat in the bath or shower. Arrange for grab rails to be fitted. Ask your social services department about this.
- Don't have trailing wires where you walk, or mats on slippery polished surfaces.
- Don't plug too many appliances into the same socket.
- Get a smoke alarm and have it fitted.
- Make sure that things you need often are stored in easily accessible places. Get a strong step-stool with a firm hand-rail.
- Keep medicines carefully. If you can't read the labels, colour code them with sticky tape. Flush no-longer-needed medicines down the lavatory.
- Have regular check-ups, especially for sight and hearing.
- Have a door-chain fitted and use it.
- Make sure your windows can be locked securely.
- Don't keep a lot of money at home.
- Ask your local housing department about help with making your home safer and more secure.

Friends and neighbours

Fortunately, most elderly people are loved and cared for by relatives and friends. Of course, nobody wants to be a nuisance to others, and most elderly people like to be as independent as possible. But this can sometimes cause problems for them. All too often an elderly person becomes cut off from society and fails to summon help when it's needed.

Those old people most in need of keeping an eye on are those who are house-bound, frail and lonely, and have no caring relatives, friends or neighbours. If you know someone in this situation, try to make sure they're not neglected.

There are so many different ways to be helpful to someone who's old. It may be no more than dropping in for a chat or offering to do some shopping. It may be cooking a meal, fetching the coal, helping them fill up a claim form, taking them to the doctor, or contacting the community care service on their behalf.

There's a large number of voluntary and statutory organisations involved in providing help and support for old people at home – anything from occupational therapists, home helps, or 'meals-on-wheels', to investment counsellors, legal advisers, helping hands and 'good companions'. The aim is to help old people lead a healthy and fulfilling life in the community.

LIFE IS FOR LIVING

We all want the best out of life, including the best of health. We know how important it is to make sure we look after ourselves and our families, and others who may need our help and support.

I hope you find this book useful in giving you the sort of advice and information that makes it easier to keep in good shape, in mind as well as body.

But I also hope that you keep the pursuit of good health in perspective. Too many people become so obsessed with healthy eating that they no longer enjoy food. Too many punish themselves with gruelling exercise regimes. Too many worry themselves sick trying to be healthy.

Life is for living, enjoying, loving and being loved – without being driven by guilt and anxiety. Life is for helping ourselves and each other find happiness, and health, because we want to, not because we feel we have to. To me the real meaning of good health is very simple, and has little to do with fitness and a long life. It's being as much in true harmony with ourselves and our fellow creatures as we possibly can. Life and health are gifts to be nurtured, enjoyed and shared.

INDEX